CSSD Dictionary
and
Reference Guide

Disclaimer

©2010 (978-1-4507-1195-1)
By the International Association of Healthcare
Central Service Materiel Management
213 West Institute Place, Suite 307
Chicago, Illinois 60610

The International Association of Healthcare
Central Service Materiel Management is a non-profit corporation.

Printed in the United States of America

ISBN 978-1-4507-1195-1

Forward

Today's healthcare industry employs professionals from many disciplines. Among them are those working in the Central Sterile Supply Department (CSSD). Like all professionals, they develop and implement a broad range of carefully considered work practices to consistently fulfill their many responsibilities.

What is a professional? The International Association of Healthcare Central Service Materiel Management (IAHCSMM) answers this question: "A professional is a person working in an occupation that requires extensive knowledge and skills to do so. A profession involves membership limited to those with education and experience in a specialized body of knowledge."

CSSD professionals must have a broad scope of knowledge about processing science. In addition, directors, managers, and supervisors in the CSSD department must know details about a variety of other subjects including human resources, financial management, and administration. How can they, often during the same work shift, resolve a highly technical sterilization issue, effectively interact with persons at higher and lower organizational levels, work on the budget, and address a facility concern by actively participating on a committee?

The ability to effectively communicate is a prerequisite for success in each task that receives the attention of each CSSD employee. Communication involves much more than just talking, listening, writing, and word processing. It also requires one to consider the goal of the communication, the person(s) who will receive the information, and the best way to organize and present (deliver) the message. In all professions, and certainly in healthcare, there is little room for "communication problems." CSSD personnel and all of their peers must be precise so they are never misunderstood.

A good command of the language of one's profession allows an individual to:

- Keep up with the fast pace of change. The ever-evolving technology of healthcare surgical procedures, instrumentation, and sterile processing brings with it a constant increase in technical terminology. An extensive vocabulary of specific terms is needed as they develop training programs, facilitate the work of staff members, contribute to process improvements, and generate alternatives to resolve problems.

- Interact with and assist customers who use highly technical terms that must be understood without exception to assure that what is needed in the surgical suites is always available when needed.

- Represent the CSSD department during interactions with internal and external constituencies and, in the process, help assure that one is an effective ambassador for the department and facility.

How to Use This Reference

The IAHCSMM CSSD Dictionary and Reference Guide is a workplace resource that you'll find useful every day. It is a reference that allows you to spend your time using information rather than searching for it.

The IAHCSMM CSSD Dictionary and Reference Guide contains a dictionary of more than 2,500 need-to-know terms that can help you to communicate more precisely and accurately. It also includes graphics of common medical symbols and conversion information for temperatures (°Fahrenheit ↔ °Centigrade) and time (24 Hour ↔ Standard) as well as information on understanding pH and more. The Dictionary of CSSD Terms within the resource you are holding has been made as useful as possible.

You'll find that using the IAHCSMM CSSD Dictionary and Reference Guide will be much faster than paging through reference manuals or doing internet searches. Another advantage: the information has been compiled and reviewed by CSSD experts.

An Accessible Resource

CSSD professionals may not spend much time in their office, but when they are there, this reference will be available. Other copies in appropriate CSSD work areas will make it convenient for others to use as well.

Employees participating in training and professional development programs will benefit from access to the information while reading and completing their other assignments. As well, those who are studying before they begin work in the CSSD profession will have a useful companion for their educational activities.

Acknowledgements and Dedication

The editors wish to acknowledge the assistance of Mr. Bruce Bird, Central Processing Manager, Primary Children's Hospital, Salt Lake City, Utah, who contributed many of the abbreviations used in this IAHCSMM CSSD Dictionary and Reference Guide. Also, a sincere "Thank You" goes to the IAHCSMM members who reviewed it:

Dewey Barker, RN, CRCST
CPD Manager
Gulf Breeze Hospital
Gulf Breeze, FL

Nola Bayes, MBA, CRCST, CIS
SPD Manager
Wentworth-Douglas Hospital
Dover, NH

Harvey Johnson, CRCST
Sterile Processing Manager
Tuality Healthcare
Hillsboro OR

Erle Shepard, CRCST, CHL, CHMMC, CIS, FCS
Central Service Manager
Centra Health
Lynchburg, VA

The editors have a great deal of confidence in the worth of the IAHCSMM CSSD Dictionary and Resource Guide and in the assistance it will provide to the CSSD profession. However, the real contributions are made by those who work in healthcare facilities protecting, serving customers and protecting patients every day. It is to them that this resource is dedicated.

Natalie Lind, CRCST, CHL, Educational Director, International Association of Healthcare Central Service Materiel Management. Moorhead, Minnesota.

Jack Ninemeier, Ph.D., The Eli Broad Graduate School of Management. Michigan State University., East Lansing, Michigan.

1   Central Service Technical Manual. Seventh Edition. Chicago, IL. International Association of Healthcare Central Service Materiel Management. 2007. (Pg. 431)

Table of Contents

Dictionary

A&P - Anterior and posterior.

AA - Affirmative action.

AAA - Abdominal aortic aneurysm.

AAMI - Association for the Advancement of Medical Instrumentation.

Abatement plan (OSHA) - A plan submitted by the healthcare facility to OSHA that details actions taken to correct a safety or health hazard violation that led to an OSHA citation.

ABC analysis – An inventory management strategy that indicates storeroom controls should first address the relatively few items with the greatest value (A items) and should lastly consider the many items with the lowest value (C items).

ABD – Abdominal.

Abdomen – The part of the body between the chest and the pelvis.

Abdominal bag - An adherent (attached) plastic pouch used to collect fluid and waste material from an abdominal stoma.

Abdominal pad (ABD pad) – A pad used over large abdominal suture sites and heavy drainage areas.

Abdominoplasty – A surgical procedure performed to flatten the abdomen by removing extra fat and skin and tightening the muscles located in the abdominal wall; commonly called "tummy tuck."

Abduction - Movement away from the midline; turning outward.

ABG - Arterial blood gas.

Ablate / Ablation - The vaporization of tissue with a laser.

ABO - A system of classifying blood groups.

Aborted (equipment) - Failed or incomplete machine cycle caused by a malfunction.

Abort - To prematurely terminate a machine cycle.

Abortion - Termination of pregnancy before the fetus is capable of survival out of the uterus.

Abrasive - Any of a wide variety of natural or manufactured gritty substances used to grind, wear down, rub away, smooth, or scour.

Abscess – An area of tissue breakdown; a localized space in the body containing pus and liquefied tissue.

Absenteeism - The extent to which employees fail to report for work when they are expected to do so.

Absolute pressure (steam sterilizer) - Gauge pressure (machine produced) + atmospheric pressure (14.7 pounds per square inch at sea level).

Absorbent towel – An all-cotton towel having a plain weave with only the warp yarns tightly twisted.

Acceptance sampling – The inspection of a sample from a larger lot to decide whether the lot should be accepted.

Account – Each healthcare organization and other organizations or businesses that are customers of a vendor.

Accountability - An obligation created when a person is delegated duties or responsibilities from higher levels of administration.

Accreditation - The process by which an organization measures the quality of its services and performance against nationally recognized standards.

Accreditation (The Joint Commission) - The accreditation decision awarded to a healthcare organization in compliance with all standards at the time of the on-site survey or that has addressed requirements for improvement in an Evidence of Standards Compliance (ESC) within 45 or 60 days following posting of the Accreditation Summary Findings Report; see also Evidence of Standards Compliance.

ACGIH - American Conference of Governmental Industrial Hygienists

Acid – A compound with a pH of less than 7.0 with a sour, sharp, or biting taste; a compound with a water solution that contains positive hydrogen ions (for example, HCl).

Acid detergent – An organic, acid-based cleaning agent; best used for removing mineral deposits.

Acid scrubber – A type of EtO emission control device.

Acid-fast bacteria - Bacteria that do not de-colorize when acid is added to the stained smear.

Acidity – The measurement of the amount of acid present.

Acidosis – The condition that results from a decrease in the pH of body fluids.

ACL - Anterior cruciate ligament.

ACLS – Advanced cardiac life support.

Acquired immune deficiency syndrome (AIDS) – A viral disease that attacks the immune system.

Acquired immunity - Immunity acquired by a person after birth.

Acquisition - The act of assuming or acquiring possession of something.

Action level - For certain chemicals, the airborne concentration of an air contaminant, calculated as an 8-hour time-weighted average, above which particular monitoring, medical surveillance, or other stated Occupational Safety and Health Administration requirements apply.

Action plan - Specific activities or lists of tasks that are part of a larger planning process such as a one-year business plan used to achieve an objective.

Acute - Short in time and relatively severe in degree.

Acute care - A type of healthcare in which a patient is treated for a short time for immediate and severe illness or injuries.

Acute disease – A disease that runs a rapid course with more or less severe symptoms.

Adaptor - A device used for connecting two parts of an apparatus.

Adduction –Movement toward the midline of the body; turning inward.

Adenoid - Glandular tissue located in the nasopharynx.

Adenoma - A tumor of glandular tissue.

Adhesion – The holding together of two surfaces or parts; a band of connective tissue between parts that are normally separate; the molecular attraction between contacting bodies.

Adhesive - Adhering, sticky, or gummed substance for the adjointment of surfaces.

Adhesive tape - A cloth, paper, or plastic strip coated on one side with an adhesive.

Adipose - Referring to fatty tissue.

Administration set - Tubing used to deliver or dispense fluids; for example, a blood or intravenous set.

Adrenal - Endocrine gland located above each kidney that produces hormones essential to life; suprarenal gland.

Advanced cardiac life support (ACLS) – Numerous types of clinical interventions for the urgent treatment of cardiac arrest and other life-threatening emergencies.

Advanced life support (ALS) - Emergency medical care for sustaining life including defibrillation, airway management, and drugs and medications.

Adverse event - A patient injury resulting from medical care or treatment.

AER – see automatic endoscope reprocessor

Aerate - To expose gas-sterilized items to warm, circulating air.

Aeration – The process by which a device is actively subjected to moving air; for example, items being sterilized with ethylene oxide gas.

Aerator (ethylene oxide) – A machine designed to speed up removal of ethylene oxide residuals from sterilized items by subjecting them to warm, circulating air.

Aerobic (bacteria) – A microorganism that requires the presence of air or oxygen for growth.

Aerosol - The suspension of ultramicroscopic solid or liquid particles in air or gas; a spray.

Affinity - Attraction.

Agar - Extract of red seaweed used as a solidifying agent in culture media.

AIDS - Acquired Immune Deficiency Syndrome; the advanced symptomatic and ultimately fatal disease in the progression of an HIV infection; see human immunodeficiency virus (HIV).

Air - The gaseous mixture that surrounds the earth which includes invisible, odorless, and tasteless gases such as oxygen and nitrogen.

Air count (bacteria) – A method of estimating the number of bacteria or microbes in a specific quantity of air.

Air exchange - The rate at which air outside an area replaces air within a given space.

Air freshener - A mechanical device or scented wick or substance used to eliminate odors.

Airborne - Suspended or carried in a gas or air stream.

Airflow (negative) - The condition that occurs when the volume of air exhausted from a room or other space is greater than the volume of air entering the room or other space.

Airflow (positive) - The condition that occurs when the volume of air entering a room or other space is greater than the volume of air exhausted from the room or other space.

Airflow regulator - A meter or gauge used to control the amount of air or other gas administered.

Airway - A rubber or plastic device inserted into the mouth or nose which reaches to the back of the throat to keep the air passageway open; may be a hollow tube or grooved device.

AKA - Above knee amputation.

Alcohol prep - Sponge saturated with isopropyl alcohol which is used to clean and disinfect the skin.

Alimentary canal – The pathway that food takes through the body's digestive system.

Alimentation - The process or act of giving or receiving nourishment.

Alkalis - Chemicals that release an excess of hydroxyl ions (OH) in a solution to yield a pH of more than 7.

Alkaline - In solution; having a pH greater than 7.

Alkalinity (of water) - A measure of how much acid water can neutralize.

Alkalosis – The condition that results from an increase in the pH of body fluids.

Alkylation – The process by which ethylene oxide destroys microorganisms resulting in the inability of a cell to normally metabolize and/or reproduce.

Allergen – A substance that causes hypersensitivity (allergy).

Allergic reaction- Caused by an allergy; the tendency to react unfavorably to a substance that is normally harmless to most people; hypersensitivity.

Allergy – The tendency to react unfavorably to a substance that is normally harmless to most people; hypersensitivity. A disorder of the immune system.

Allocate - The act of determining the amount of money to be spent on an expense for which the CSSD department is responsible.

ALS – Advanced life support.

Alternative dispute resolution (ADR) - A voluntary procedure to resolve disputes or conflicts between individuals, groups, or labor and management in which a neutral third party facilitates discussion and assists the parties in reaching a binding agreement.

Alveolus (pl. alveoli) - One of millions of tiny air sacs in the lungs through which gases are exchanged between the outside air and the blood; also tooth socket.

Ambient air - Air in an uncontrolled environment; for example, outside air.

Ambient condition - Environmental conditions such as pressure, temperature, and humidity which are normal for a specific location.

Ambu bag – See bag valve mask.

Ambulatory care (outpatient care) - Healthcare services provided without admitting the patient to the hospital.

Ambulatory Surgical Procedures - Surgery performed on an outpatient basis. It may be hospital-based or performed in an office or surgicenter.

Ameba (pl. amebas) - Protozoon that moves by extruding finger-like elements (pseudopods); also spelled amoeba (pl. amoebae).

Amebiasis - Infection with pathogenic amebas; acute amebiasis is called amebic dysentery.

American National Standards Institute (ANSI) - A national organization that oversees the creation, promotion, and use of voluntary standards for many United States industries including healthcare.

Amino acid – A building block of protein; organic chemical compounds containing an amino group and a carboxyl group which form the chief structure of proteins.

Amitosis - Direct cell division.

Amniocentesis - Removal of fluid and cells from the amniotic sac for prenatal diagnostic tests.

Amniotic fluid – The fluid that surrounds the fetus.

Amniotic sac – The fluid-filled sac that surrounds and cushions the developing fetus.

Amoeboid movement – The crawling movement of cells that occurs as the cell successively becomes longer and then retracts.

Amputation - A surgical procedure involving the removal of all or part of a body limb generally performed to control pain or a disease process in the affected limb such as gangrene or a malignancy.

Anaerobe (bacteria) – A microorganism that grows only or best in the absence of oxygen.

Anal - Relating to the anus, the rectal opening on the body surface.

Analgesic - Relieving pain; a pain-relieving agent that does not cause loss of consciousness.

Analysis - A thorough examination of an issue or process.

Anaphylaxis – The state of hypersensitivity to a protein resulting from a previous introduction of the protein into the body that can result in death without treatment.

Anastomosis – The surgical or pathological formation of a passage between two normally distinct structures such as tubular organs.

Anatomy – The study of body structure.

Ancillary services - Supplemental healthcare services including laboratory, radiology, and physical therapy services provided during a patient's hospital stay.

Anemia - Reduction in the amount of red cells or hemoglobin in the blood resulting in inadequate delivery of oxygen to the tissues.

Anesthesia - Loss of sensation (particularly of pain).

Anesthesiologist - A physician specializing in the medical study and application of anesthetics; see anesthetic.

Anesthetic - An agent that produces anesthesia which can be general and produce sound sleep or local and render a specific area insensitive to pain.

Anesthetist – A person trained to administer anesthetics.

Aneurysm – A blood vessel abnormality characterized by a weakening of the wall of an artery that leads to a "ballooning" of the vessel wall which forms a sac filled with blood.

Angina - Severe choking pain; a disease or condition producing such pain.

Angina pectoris – A suffocating pain in the chest usually caused by lack of oxygen supply to the heart.

Angio catheter - An intravenous catheter used for the administration of intravenous fluids.

Angiogram – The introduction of a contrast material (radiopaque dye) into the blood vessels for an x-ray photograph.

Angstrom – The unit of measure for visible light.

Anhydrous - Containing no water.

Animate - Having life.

Anion – A negatively charged particle (ion).

Anionic – A compound with a negative electrical charge on the large organic portion of the molecule which is relatively hydrophobic and lipophilic; used as a synthetic detergent.

Ankle support - An elasticized cloth support used to stabilize a sprained or injured ankle.

Anorexia - Loss of appetite.

Anoscope - A small medical viewing scope inserted into the anus to allow visualization of the anus and the lower portion of the rectum; commonly used to identify abnormalities such as inflammation, hemorrhoids, or tumors.

Anoxia - Lack of oxygen.

ANSI - American National Standards Institute.

ANT – Anterior.

Antagonist – A muscle with an action opposite that of a given movement; a substance that opposes the action of another substance.

Anterior - Toward the front or belly surface; ventral.

Anterior & posterior repair (A&P) - The repair of a cystocele (anterior) or rectocele (posterior).

Anterior repair - The repair of a cystocele: a herniation of the bladder wall into the vagina which sometimes occurs after childbirth.

Anthrax - Infectious disease of cattle and sheep caused by a spore-forming bacterium (Bacillus anthracis) which may be transmitted to man through handling of infected products.

Antibacterial - Destroying or stopping the growth of bacteria.

Antibacterial serum – An antiserum that destroys or prevents the growth of bacteria.

Antibiotic – A substance produced by one microorganism that will kill or inhibit another microorganism.

Antibody – A protein produced in the body which reacts against a specific foreign molecule (antigen).

Anticoagulant – An agent that prevents blood coagulation.

Anti-embolism (support hose) - Elastic support hose sized to a patient that is used to prevent clotting of blood by maintaining continuous pressure on the legs.

Antigen – A substance which causes the body to produce antibodies.

Antiseptic – A solution which inhibits the growth of bacteria; usually used topically and only on animate objects.

Antiserum – A serum containing antibodies given to provide passive immunity.

Antitoxin – An immune serum which neutralizes the action of a toxin.

Anus - Lower opening of the alimentary canal.

Anvil - One of the three middle ear bones; attaches to the hammer and stirrup.

AORN - The Association of periOperative Registered Nurses.

Aorta – The largest blood vessel in the body.

Aortogram tray - A set of instruments and supplies necessary for introduction of a contrast material (radiopaque dye) into the aorta for an x-ray photograph.

A&P – Anterior and posterior repair.

APIC - Association for Professionals in Infection Control and Epidemiology, Inc.

Appendectomy - Removal of the appendix.

Applicant files - Application forms and resumes maintained by an employer and used during the employee selection process.

Applicant pool - All persons who submitted an employment application for a specific position.

Application (computer) - A computer program that performs work not related to the computer; examples include word processing and spreadsheets.

Applicator - A wooden, plastic, or metal stick with an absorbent tip used for applying a substance.

Aquathermia - Application of warm or cold water for therapy.

Aquathermia control unit - A unit containing distilled water powered by an electrical motor with a temperature gauge on one side and two coupling outlets at the base that attach to a pad that has recirculating coils; the unit continuously heats distilled water and pumps it through the pad.

Aqueous - Water; prepared with water.

Aqueous humor – The watery-like fluid between the cornea and the eye lens.

Aqueous solution - Liquid in which a chemical substance is dissolved in water.

Arbitration - A mini-trial used by parties to resolve a dispute held in an effort to avoid a court trial.

Arbitration (compulsory) - An action in which an arbitrator is appointed to make a binding decision on parties negotiating a contact.

Arbitration (voluntary) - An action in which parties submit a dispute to an external disinterested third party for binding or non-binding resolution after presentation of evidence and related discussion.

Architect - A licensed professional who focuses on the aesthetic design of buildings and spaces, structures, mechanical systems, acoustics, regulatory, and other requirements needed to make buildings useful and safe for their occupancy.

Arteriole - The vessel between a small artery and a capillary.

Arm board - A flat piece of wood, plastic, or metal used to stabilize an arm at the wrist or elbow to promote the administration of blood or intravenous feedings.

Arrhythmia - Abnormal rhythm of the heartbeat.

Arteries - Vessels that carry blood away from the heart.

Arterial blood gas (ABG) – A test that measures the levels of oxygen and carbon dioxide in the blood to determine how well the lungs are working.

Arteriogram - An x-ray of blood vessels which can be seen after an injection of a dye that shows up in the x-ray pictures.

Arteriogram tray - A set of instruments and supplies necessary to inject a contrast medium (radiopaque dye) into the bloodstream for an x-ray photograph.

Arteriosclerosis - Hardening of the arteries.

Artery - A blood vessel that carries oxygenated blood from the heart to the tissues.

Arthritis - Inflammation of the joints.

Arthrogram - The injection of a contrast medium (radiopaque dye) into a joint for an x-ray photograph.

Arthroplasty - A generic term for any joint surgery designed to restore joint function. A prosthetic device is often used to replace the native joint totally or partially. A total arthroplasty involves prosthetic replacement of both sides of a joint, and a hemiarthroplasty involves replacement of only one side of a joint such as a hip bipolar prosthesis.

Ascending aortic aneurysm - An aortic aneurysm is an enlargement of a weakened area of the aorta; those that involve the ascending aorta are called thoracic aortic aneurysms.

Asepsis – The absence of microorganisms that cause disease.

Asepsis (surgical) - Procedures to eliminate the presence of all microorganisms and/or to prevent the introduction of microorganisms to an area.

Aseptic - Free from pathogenic organisms; a means of preventing infection.

Aseptic technique – An activity or procedure that prevents infection or breaks the chain of infection.

Asepto syringe - A glass or plastic syringe with an attached bulb used for aspiration, irrigation, and feeding.

ASHD - Atherosclerotic heart disease.

Asphyxia – The condition caused by lack of oxygen in inspired air.

Aspirate - To draw by suction; examples: when fluid is removed with a syringe, and when material is drawn into the lungs during inspiration.

Aspirating tubes - Tubes used to obtain and collect fluids for a specimen.

Aspiration – The act of drawing in by suction.

Aspirator - A device or instrument that removes fluids or gases from a space by suction; a suction pump used medically to evacuate a body cavity.

Asset - Something of value owned by an organization or person.

Asset (current) – An asset that is expected to be used within one year.

Association for the Advancement of Medical Instrumentation (AAMI) – A voluntary organization that develops Recommended Practices and Standards that are considered major resources for Central Service guidelines.

Association for Professionals in Infection Control and Epidemiology, Inc. (APIC). A voluntary organization that addresses the prevention and control of infections and related outcomes.

Association of periOperative Registered Nurses (AORN) – A voluntary organization that develops nationally recognized Standards, Recommended Practices, and Guidelines for the periOperative setting.

Atherosclerosis - Hardening of the arteries caused by deposits of yellowish, fat-like material on blood vessel linings.

Atherosclerotic heart disease (ASHD) - A heart disease caused by the lowering of blood supply to the heart muscle due to narrowing of the cavity of one or both coronary arteries; caused by accumulation of fatty material on the inner lining of the arterial wall; also called ischemic heart disease and coronary heart disease.

Athletic supporter - Elastic support for the male genitals; also called "jockstrap."

Atomizer - A device used to produce a fine spray; nebulizer.

Atria - The two upper chambers of the heart.

Atraumatic - not producing injury or damage. Used to describe instruments and devices that are unlikely to cause tissue damage.

Atrial fibrillation (AFIB) - An irregular and often rapid heart rate that commonly causes poor blood flow to the body.

Atrial flutter (AFL) – A condition similar to atrial fibrillation in which the upper chambers (atria) of the heart beat too fast.

Atrium - One of the two upper chambers of the heart.

Atrophy - Wasting or decrease in size of a part.

Attendance policy - A written departmental or facility requirement that employees must be on time and present during scheduled shifts.

Attenuated – To weaken.

Attitude - The positive or negative feelings, beliefs, and values about something such as people, situations, or objects that influences a person to act in certain ways.

Attrition - The loss of employees from voluntary and involuntary terminations, deaths, and retirements.

Atrioventricular (AV) - Pertaining to the atria (the upper chambers of the heart) and the ventricles (the lower chambers of the heart).

Audit trail – A chronological (step-by-step) record that allows financial data to be traced to its source. Example for a medical supply would include purchase order—delivery invoice—check number used for payment of the delivery invoice.

Austenitic (stainless steel) - Non-magnetic stainless steel that cannot be heat-hardened and which is more corrosion-resistant than martensitic stainless steel; also called 300 series stainless steel.

Authority - Power; the ability to do something including making decisions.

Authorized signature - A signature on a purchasing document made by someone authorized to represent the facility.

Autoclave - Equipment that uses steam under pressure to sterilize, usually at temperatures of 250° or 270°F (121°C or 132°C).

Autoclave film - A continuous roll of paper or transparent plastic tubing used for packaging items for steam sterilization.

Autoclave tape - Tape printed with ink sensitized for heat and moisture used for packaging items for stream sterilization. The ink changes to a dark color during the sterilization process (external indicator).

Autocratic (leadership style) - A leadership approach in which decisions are typically made and problems are resolved without input from affected staff members.

Auto-logon - A system that enables a user to gain access to a computer system without user intervention; also call "auto-login."

Automated guided vehicle (AGV) - A mobile robot device guided by markers or wires in the floor, optical vision, or scanners that is used to transport materials in a warehouse.

Automated supply replenishment system – A replenishment system in which items removed from inventory are automatically identified and tracked. When a reorder point is reached, item information is generated on a supply pick list in the central storeroom. Items are then issued and transferred to the appropriate user area.

Automatic - A self-acting or self-regulating mechanism.

Automatic endoscope reprocessor (AER) - Automated machine designed to clean, disinfect, and rinse flexible endoscopes.

Autonomic nervous system – The part of the nervous system that controls smooth muscle, cardiac muscle, and glands; the motor portion of the visceral or involuntary nervous system.

Autopsy - Examination of a dead body to evaluate the presence of disease or the cause of death.

AV – Atrioventricular; Atriovenous.

Axilla - Hollow beneath the arm where it joins the body; armpit.

Axillary - Pertaining to or located near the armpit.

Axillary dissection - Surgery to remove lymph nodes under the arm.

B

Bacillus (pl., bacilli) - Rod-shaped bacteria; a genus of the family Bacillaceae.

Bacillus atrophaeus - Resistant microorganism used to challenge Ethylene Oxide sterilizers; formerly called Bacillus subtilis.

Bacillus of Calmette-Guerin (BCG) - Vaccine against tuberculosis made from a bovine strain of tubercle bacilli attenuated through long culturing.

Bacillus stearothermophilus - See geobacillus stearothermophilus.

Bacillus subtilis - See Bacillus atrophaeus.

Back door selling (purchasing policy) – The act of a vendor attempting to contact or influence a user department employee without approval of the purchasing department.

Background check - The process of verifying job applicant information that may include contacting former employers, obtaining educational records, and requesting criminal or consumer credit reports.

Back-order - The situation in which a product normally available in a vendor's inventory is out of stock and has been ordered from the vendor's own product source.

Bacteremia – A condition in which bacteria are in the bloodstream.

Bacteria (sing. bacterium) - Single-celled, plant-like microbes that reproduce by splitting; some cause diseases; also called "germs."

Bacterial count - Method of estimating the number of bacteria in a sample unit.

Bactericidal - Relating to the destruction of bacteria.

Bactericide – A substance that kills bacteria.

Bacteriology – The science of the study of bacteria.

Bacteriophage – A virus that parasitizes and multiplies exclusively in bacteria.

Bacteriostasis – The condition in which bacterial growth is inhibited, but the organisms are not killed.

Bacteriostat – A substance that inhibits the growth of bacteria.

Bacteriostatic – The inhibition of bacterial growth without their destruction.

Bag valve mask (BVM) - A hand-held device that provides positive pressure ventilation to someone who is not breathing or breathing inadequately; also called ambu bag.

Balance sheet – A financial summary of what a healthcare facility owns (assets), owes (liabilities), and is worth (equity) at a specific point in time; example: the last day of every month.

Ballpark - A slang term meaning an estimated amount.

Bandage - Fabric or gauze used as a protective covering for a wound or other injury.

Band-Aid – The trade name for an adhesive bandage with a gauze pad in the center that is used as a protection for minor wounds.

Bar code - Numerous machine-readable rectangular bars and spaces arranged in a specific way to represent the numbers, letters, and other symbols used to identify a product.

Bariatric - The branch of medicine that deals with the causes, prevention, and treatment of obesity, both pharmacological and surgical. Bariatric medical furniture such as bariatric chairs and tables are designed to accommodate the special needs of overweight or obese people.

Barium sulfate - A fine white powder that becomes bulky when mixed with water and is used as an opaque medium for x-ray examination of the digestive tract.

Barrier - Anything that prevents or obstructs passage.

Barrier cloth - Fabrics made of blends of cotton/polyester designed specifically to provide a bacterial barrier.

Barrier properties - Ability of a material to resist the penetration of liquids and/or microorganisms.

Basal ganglia - Gray masses in the lower part of the forebrain that assist with muscle coordination.

Base – A compound with a pH above 7.0.

Basin - An open, rounded vessel used for holding water and other fluids.

BCG - Bacillus of Calmette-Guerin; a tuberculosis vaccine.

Bed board - A wooden or plastic device the length and width of a mattress that is placed on top of bedsprings under the mattress to provide very firm support; used to treat back problems.

Bed check control unit – A device that sounds an alarm when a patient gets out of bed; also called bed check device.

Bedpan - A metal or plastic receptacle used for receiving urine and feces from a patient confined to bed.

Bedsore - Decubitus ulcer; an ulcer-like pressure sore over a body area due to prolonged confinement in bed or continuous pressure that limits the nutrition of the affected area.

Behavior modification - Efforts to change or eliminate an individual's undesirable behavior by specifying expected behavior.

Behavioral interviewing - The process of asking job applicants open-ended questions during applicant selection, performance appraisal, and other interviews to generate information that identifies previous reactions to specific situations; also called behavioral-based interviewing; see open-ended question.

Behavioral risk management - A method of analyzing and identifying workplace behavioral issues and implementing policies and programs to correct or eliminate specific employee behavioral problems.

Bench trial - A trial held before a judge sitting without a jury.

Benchmark - A standard to compare and improve one's own products or services by measuring them against specified standards.

Benchmarking - Activities to identify and analyze best practices to discover areas of and processes for performance improvement.

Benchmarking (external) - Activities to analyze work processes used by Central Service departments in other healthcare facilities.

Benchmarking (internal) - Activities to undertake a performance analysis of processes used within the same organization: between departments, between work areas within the same department, and between the same departments in different facilities within a multi-facility organization.

Benchmarking database system – Measureable standards that can be used for performance baselines within an industry.

Benchmarking indicators - Measurable indicators used to benchmark the performance of a CSS department; examples include instrument assembly accuracy and productivity data.

Benefits - Indirect financial compensation to attract and retain employees and/or to comply with legal mandates.

Benign - A tumor that does not spread and is not recurrent or becoming worse; not malignant.

Benzoin - A balsamic resin used as a local antiseptic; a stimulant to promote healing; a protective coating for decubitus ulcers; an expectorant; and an inhalant used in steamers for treating respiratory disorders.

Bereavement leave - A policy providing a specified number of paid days-off to enable an employee to attend funeral services for an employee's spouse, parent, child, grandparent, sibling, or in-law.

Best practice - An activity or procedure that has been successful in another situation and that might be the best way to do something in one's own organization.

Betadine - Trade name for povidone-iodine preparations; used for antiseptic purposes such as hand washes and surgical scrubs and preps.

Bevel - Angle at which the point of a needle or blade is ground.

Bid – Price quotation, as in "The vendor bid (submitted a price quotation of) $17.12 for the item."

Bid (competitive) – The act of sending requests for price quotations to more than one vendor with the goal of receiving a lower price from one vendor for a supply item or service of agreed-upon quality; see RFQ.

Bidding (human resources) - The internal posting of position vacancies to enable current employees to apply before the employer seeks qualified candidates through external recruitment.

Bilateral - Affecting the right and left side of body.

Bilateral salpingo-oophorectomy (BSO) - A surgical procedure to remove the ovaries and fallopian tubes.

Bile – A substance produced in the liver that emulsifies fats.

Bile bag – A plastic pouch used to collect bile following gallbladder surgery.

Bili lights (phototherapy) - Specialty lights that treat infants with jaundice: a yellow coloring of the skin and eyes related to abnormal liver function.

Binary fission – The typical method of bacterial reproduction in which a cell divides into two equal parts.

Binder - A large band of cloth or elastic worn around the abdomen or chest for support; types of binders include abdominal-elastic, scultetus, breast, chest, and t-binders.

Bio - Word element meaning life or living.

Biobarrier - A package system that allows a sterilant to enter a pack and, after sterilization, creates a barrier to contamination. Biobarriers protect sterile items from contamination, but they are not impenetrable. Special storage and handling protocols are required to ensure sterility.

Bioburden – The number of microorganisms on a contaminated object; also called bioload or microbial load.

Biocidal - The ability to kill microorganisms.

Biodegradable - Readily decomposed by bacteria or enzymatic actions.

Biofilm – A matrix that contains living and dead cells and a polysaccharide that is exuded by microorganisms when they grow in water or water solutions or in vivo (example: the bloodstream). Biofilm prevents antimicrobial agents such as sterilants, disinfectants, and antibiotics from reaching microorganisms.

Biohazard signage - Notices in easily-seen locations that alert persons about the presence of harmful bacteria, viruses, or other dangerous biohazardous agents or organisms.

Biohazardous - Relating to infectious agents that present a risk or potential risk to human health either directly through infections or indirectly through the environment.

Biological - Relating to biology.

Biological indicator (BI) – A sterilization process monitoring device consisting of a standardized, viable population of microorganisms (usually bacterial spores) known to be resistant to the mode of sterilization being monitored.

Biological transfer of infection – The mode of transfer of infection from host to host by an animal or insect in which the disease-causing agent goes through a development cycle.

Biology – The science which studies living things, both animals and plants.

Biomedical engineer - A person professionally trained in biotechnology and the repair and maintenance of biomedical equipment.

Biomedical engineering department – The hospital department that performs safety inspections and function tests on medical equipment; frequently abbreviated "Biomed Department."

Biomedical technician (BMET) - A person trained in the technical aspects of repair and maintenance of biomedical equipment.

Biopsy (bx) – The removal of tissue or other material from the living body for examination, usually under the microscope.

Biopsy needle - Needle used for the extraction of tissue for microscopic examination.

Biotechnology - The engineering and biological study of human beings as related to machines.

Bipolar electrocautery – A type of electrocautery in which the active and receiving electrodes are both placed at the site of cauterization. The probe is usually in the shape of a forceps with each tine forming one electrode so only the tissue between the electrodes is cauterized; also called diathermy.

BKA - Below knee amputation.

Bladder - A membranous sac, especially the urinary bladder, that serves as the receptacle for a liquid.

Bladder irrigation - The washing of the urinary bladder with cleansing or therapeutic solutions.

Blakemore esophageal tube - A tube with an inflatable balloon used to control esophageal hemorrhaging.

Blanket order - A pre-negotiated agreement covering a specific time period (example: six months) about the price and/or quantity of products to be delivered during that time period.

Blended workforce - A workforce comprised of permanent full-time, part-time, and temporary employees.

Blocking - The process of obstructing or deadening.

Blood - Connective tissue fluid that transports many substances throughout the circulatory system.

Blood administration set - A special tubing used to dispense blood products to a patient.

Blood bank – A place where blood is typed, tested, and stored until it is needed for transfusion.

Blood collection set - A special tubing used to extract and collect blood.

Blood gas tray - A collection of supplies and equipment necessary to determine the oxygen and carbon dioxide levels in the blood.

Blood pressure - Pressure exerted on the blood vessels by blood.

Blood pressure cuff - A secured band positioned on an arm above the elbow with tubing attached to a sphygmomanometer; used to apply pressure against an artery to measure the blood pressure of the artery wall.

Blood pump – A cuff with a hand pump used for rapid infusion of blood.

Bloodborne pathogen standards (OSHA) - Regulations issued by the Occupational Safety and Health Administration that relate to occupational exposure to blood or other potentially infectious materials.

Bloodborne pathogens - Microorganisms that are present in human blood and can produce disease in humans.

Blow bottle - Container used for intermittent positive pressure exercises for the lungs.

BLS - Basic life support.

Board of Directors - Persons who sit as a governing body and take responsibility for an organization's management.

Board of Trustees - A committee or governing body responsible for managing and holding the trust funds, assets, or property belonging to others; example: the top-level governing board for a public hospital.

Body language - Non-verbal communication by movement of one's body.

Body restraint - A device such as a belt, vest, or net used to safely immobilize a patient.

Boil (heating) - To heat a fluid to the point of bubbling and turning the fluid into a gaseous state.

Boil (skin) - A pus-filled, painful swelling of the skin and subcutaneous tissue caused by bacterial infection; also called furuncle.

Bone forceps - Strong forceps used for seizing or removing fragments of bone.

Bone marrow - The soft, sponge-like material in the cavities of bones made up of blood vessels, connective tissue, fat, and blood-producing cells.

Bone marrow needle - Needle used to extract marrow from a bone for examination.

Bone plate - A thin metal implant used to immobilize bone segments that is affixed with screws to properly align the bone and aid in the healing process.

Bone screw - A metal implant inserted into the bone that is used to immobilize fractured bone segments to aid in the healing process; also used as an adjunct to spine fusion surgery to help hold implants in place.

Borosilicate - Alkaline-free silicate glass having at least 5% boric oxide and used especially in heat resistant glassware; a very hard glass (Pyrex).

Bottleneck (process) - The problem that arises when input occurs faster than the next step can use it to create output. Example: case carts arrive in the decontamination area faster than they can be processed.

Botulism - Food poisoning caused by the toxin of an anaerobic, spore-forming bacterium (clostridium botulinum) in contaminated canned or smoked foods.

Boundaryless organization - An organization that removes roadblocks to maximize information flow. Its goals include developing greater flexibility and responsiveness to change and encouraging the free flow of information and ideas throughout the organization.

Bowel - Intestine; the digestive tract below the stomach.

Bowie-Dick test - A test run daily to validate the vacuum function of a steam sterilizer. The test should be run in an empty load and at the same time of the day each day.

Box lock – The point where the two jaws or blades of an instrument connect and pivot.

BP - Blood pressure

Brain - Main control unit of the central nervous system.

Brain stem - Controls many automatic body functions such as heartbeat and breathing.

Brainstorm - A group problem solving or alternative generation tactic in which all group members suggest possible ideas.

Breast binder - A supportive band of cloth or elastic device that holds the breasts firmly in proper position; used postpartum and postoperatively.

Breast prosthesis - An internal or external replacement of, or addition to, a breast by an artificial substitute.

Breast pump - A mechanical device used to extract and collect milk from the breast.

Breast reduction – A typically outpatient surgical procedure that involves the removal of fat, excess breast tissue, and skin, resulting in a smaller breast size; also called "reduction mammoplasty."

Broad-spectrum - Term indicating that an antibiotic is effective against a large array of microorganisms.

Bronchi - Tubes extending from the trachea into both sides of the lungs.

Bronchiole - One of the small bronchial subdivisions that branch throughout the lungs.

Bronchoscopy - A test that permits the doctor to see the breathing passages through a lighted scope.

BSO - Bilateral salpingo-opherectomy.

Budget - A detailed plan for generating revenue, if applicable, and incurring expenses for the CSS department; also called departmental operating budget.

Budget (zero-based) - An approach to budget preparation that requires planners to justify all expenses. When used, the CSSD leader plans for each new fiscal period beginning with zero dollars, and budget planners must justify the entire amount budgeted for the new period.

Buffer – A substance that prevents sharp changes in the pH of a solution.

Bulb syringe – A rubber or plastic syringe used for suctioning and irrigating ears or the nasal and oral cavities of infants; also called asepto syringe.

Bullying (workplace) - The repeated, health-harming mistreatment of one or more persons (targets) by one or more persons; examples include verbal abuse, offensive conduct, and work interference.

Bumping - A slang term referring to the practice that allows employees with seniority whose positions have been eliminated to assume a position for which they are qualified that is currently occupied by someone with less seniority.

Bureaucratic (leadership style) - A leadership approach that involves "management by the book" and the enforcement of policies, procedures, and rules.

Bursa – A small, fluid-filled sac in an area subject to stress around bones and joints.

Business case - A formal report that addresses the need for a project, its expected benefits, anticipated costs, and estimated return on investment, among other factors, to justify the required expenditure.

Business plan - A plan that indicates what facility or CSSD personnel will do within the next year to move toward the goals identified in the facility's or department's long-range plan.

Butterfly anal dressing – A butterfly-shaped, moist, medicated gauze dressing dispensed from a jar that is used for anal cleansing and analgesia in anal surgery.

Butterfly infusion set - A scalp vein set; short intravenous catheter with tubing used for intravenous fluid administration.

Buyers (qualified) – Persons with the authority to make purchase decisions for a healthcare facility; also called a Purchasing Agent

BVM – Bag valve mask.

Bx – Biopsy.

Bypass - A surgical procedure in which the doctor creates a new pathway for the flow of body fluids.

C

C – Centigrade; Celsius.

CAB – Coronary artery bypass.

CABG -- Coronary artery bypass graft.

CAD – Coronary artery disease.

Cadaver - A dead body usually intended for dissection.

Caesarean section - See cesarean section.

Calcium gluconate - A compound used in solution to replenish calcium in the body.

Calibration – The comparison of a measurement system or device of unknown accuracy to a national standard of known accuracy to detect, correlate, report, or adjust any variation from the required performance limits of the unverified measurement system or device.

Call back roster – A listing of each staff member's telephone number that is used to inform employees to report to work in an emergency.

Cancellous bone screw - A type of bone screw with a smooth shank proximally and coarse threads distally designed to be inserted into cancellous bone in such a way that the threads do not cross a fracture line.

Cancer – The uncontrolled growth of a tumor that spreads to other tissue; a malignant neoplasm.

Cannulas - Surgical instruments with a hollow barrel (lumen) through their center; often inserted for drainage.

Capillaries - Vessels that connect veins and arteries.

Capital budget – A financial plan for acquisition of new and replacement equipment and other fixed assets and for facility remodeling or construction; see fixed assets.

Capital equipment - Item of major importance; usually defined by a set dollar amount and which is depreciated over the useful life of the equipment rather than being expensed at purchase.

Capital expenditure – The cost to acquire a long-term asset such as a building, property, or equipment or to make major improvements on a long-term asset.

Capsule (microorganism) – A gelatinous, colorless envelope or slime layer surrounding the cell wall of certain microorganisms.

Carbohydrate – A simple sugar or compound made from simple sugars linked together.

Carbon dioxide – A gaseous waste product of cellular metabolism; abbreviated CO_2.

Carcinogen – Any substance that produces cancer.

Carcinogenic - Having the ability to produce or cause cancer.

Carcinoma - Malignant growth of epithelial cells; a form of cancer.

Cardiac arrest - Sudden and often unexpected stoppage of the heartbeat.

Cardiologist - A physician who specializes in cardiology; see cardiology.

Cardiology - The study of the heart and its functions and diseases.

Cardiopulmonary resuscitation (CPR) – A method to restore heartbeat and breathing by mouth-to-mouth resuscitation and closed chest cardiac massage.

Cardiovascular - Pertaining to the heart and blood vessels.

Carditis - Inflammation of the heart; myocarditis.

Career ladder – A plan projecting progressively more responsible professional positions that serves as a foundation for a professional development program.

Caries - Tooth decay; also called cavities.

C-arm - A type of radiologic equipment so named because of its C-shaped arc surrounding its table. This x-ray image intensifier is normally used for either plain fluoroscopy or digital subtraction angiography (DSA), and it allows for lower x-ray doses to be used on patients by magnifying the intensity produced in the output image so the viewer can easily see the structure of the object being imaged.

C-arm table - A table for examination used in conjunction with an x-ray image intensifier that allows for the placement of the C-shaped arc of the x-ray image intensifier that arcs over the top and bottom of the table; see C-arm.

Carotid angiogram - The injection of radiopaque dye into the bloodstream to observe the blood circulation to the brain by means of x-rays.

Carotid artery - Either of two principal arteries of the neck that carry blood to the head.

Carpal - Refers to the bones in the wrist.

Carpal tunnel syndrome – Pressure on the median nerve in the wrist that supplies feeling and movement to parts of the hand.

Carrier – An individual who harbors and disseminates specific pathogenic microorganisms without manifesting clinical symptoms and who serves as an intermediary in the transfer of diseases to a susceptible person.

Cartilage – A type of flexible connective tissue.

Case cart – An inventory control system for products and equipment typically used in the operating room. An enclosed cart is generally prepared for one surgical case and is not used for general supply replenishment; also called case cart system.

Case cart pull sheet (pick list) – A list of specific supplies, utensils, and instruments used to assemble the items needed for individual surgical procedures.

Case management – The coordination and review of a patient's treatment to achieve the desired health outcome in a cost-effective manner. Case managers coordinate healthcare delivery including appropriate referral to consultants, specialists, hospitals, and ancillary providers.

Case manager – A healthcare professional who coordinates services and involvement of all interested parties including patients, providers, agencies, and insurers to provide patients with an appropriate care plan.

Case mix – The different types of patients treated within a specific hospital. Patient classification systems like Diagnostic Related Groupings (DRGs) can be used to measure a hospital's case mix.

Case study – A training method that presents a real-world situation and allows trainees to apply what was learned in their training to address the identified problem(s).

Casual employment – The practice of hiring employees on an as-needed basis to substitute for permanent full-time employees on short- and long-term absences or to meet additional staffing needs during peak workloads. Casual employees do not receive benefits.

CAT - Computed axial tomography.

Catalyst – A substance which influences the speed of a chemical reaction without being consumed.

Cataract - Opacity of the eye lens or lens capsule.

Catheter – A slender, flexible tube of rubber, plastic, or metal used for draining a body cavity or injecting fluids through a body passage.

Catheter care kit - A set of instruments and supplies used to clean the genitalia surrounding an in-dwelling urinary catheter.

Catheter guide - An instrument used to direct catheters into position in the body cavity.

Catheter irrigation tray - A set of instruments and supplies used for the cleansing of a canal such as the urinary bladder.

Catheterization - The introduction of a catheter into a body passageway.

Catheterization laboratory (cath lab) – An examination room with diagnostic imaging equipment to support catheterization procedures.

Cation – A positively charged particle (ion).

Cation resin tank – A tank into which untreated hard water flows and in which sodium ions are exchanged for calcium and magnesium ions to produce soft water.

Cationic – A compound containing a positive electrical charge on the large organic hydrophobic molecule which exhibits germicidal properties.

Cat scan - See computed axial tomography.

Caucus - A term relating to the suspension of negotiations so both sides can reconsider their positions.

Caudal anesthesia - A regional anesthesia used in childbirth. An anesthetic agent is injected into the caudal area of the spine via the lower end of the sacrum to deaden nerves affecting the cervix, vagina, and perineum.

Causative agent (chain of infection) – A microorganism that causes an infectious disease.

Caustic - A corrosive and burning agent, particularly an alkali that will destroy living tissue.

Cauterization - The act of coagulating blood and destroying tissue with heat, caustic agent, or by freezing.

Cautery - Burner; a means of destroying tissue by electricity, heat, or corrosive chemicals. Thermocautery consists of a red hot or white hot object, usually a wire or pointed metallic instrument, heated in a flame or with electricity.

Cavitation – The process used by an ultrasonic cleaner in which low-pressure bubbles in a cleaning solution burst inward to dislodge soil from instruments.

CBC - Complete blood count.

cc – Cubic centimeter.

CCU – Coronary care unit.

CDC – Centers for Disease Control and Prevention.

Cecum - Small pouch at the beginning of the large intestine.

Ceiling limit (CL) - According to OSHA: "The employee's exposure to an air contaminant which shall not be exceeded during any part of the work day. If instantaneous monitoring is not feasible, then the ceiling shall be assessed as a 15-minute time-weighted average exposure which shall not be exceeded at any time over a working day;" see threshold limit value.

Cell - The basic unit of life; the smallest structural unit of living organisms capable of performing all basic life functions.

Cell membrane - The outer covering of a cell that regulates what enters and leaves the cell.

Cellulitis - The diffuse inflammation of connective tissues.

Celsius - A temperature scale having the freezing point of water at 0° (degrees) and boiling point at 100° (degrees) developed by Anders Celsius; also called Centigrade.

Centers for Disease Control and Prevention (CDC) – An agency of the U.S. Department of Health and Social Services whose privacy function is to investigate outbreaks of and control diseases.

Centers for Medicare and Medicaid Services (CMS) – A federal agency within the U.S. Department of Health and Human Services responsible for Medicare, Medicaid, State Children's Health Insurance Program (SCHIP), and the Health Insurance Portability and Accountability Act (HIPPA).

Centigrade – See Celsius.

Central nervous system (CNS) – The part of the nervous system that includes the brain and spinal cord.

Central processing unit (CPU) – The part of a computer system that carries out the instructions of a computer program.

Central Sterile Supply Department (CSSD) - The department that processes, stores, and distributes medical and surgical supplies and equipment; also called Central Service Department and Supply Processing Distribution Department.

Central Service Department – See Central Sterile Supply Department (CSSD).

Central venous pressure (CVP) – A direct measurement of the blood pressure in the thoracic vena cava near the right atrium.

Central venous pressure (CVP) set - A device used to measure pressure within the veins.

Centralization - The process of consolidating all activity under one central group or location. Example: most healthcare facilities centralize sterile processing activities.

Centralized patient order entry (CPOE) – An electronic system that allows users in different departments to order items from other departments with associated charges being applied to specific patients.

Centrifuge – A device used to spin test tubes; used in the laboratory.

Cerebellum – The second largest part of the brain that controls muscle coordination, body balance, and posture.

Cerebral aneurysm – The abnormal bulging of the walls of a blood vessel which supply blood to the brain. Over time, the blood pressure inside the aneurysm can lead to its expansion and eventual rupture; commonly called brain aneurysm.

Cerebrospinal fluid (CSF) - Fluid that circulates in and around the brain and spinal cord.

Cerebrovascular accident (CVA) – A condition involving bleeding from the brain or obstruction of blood flow to brain tissue, usually resulting from hypertension or atherosclerosis; also called stroke.

Cerebrum – The largest part of the brain that controls mental activities and movement.

Cervical - Referring to the neck; a neck-like part of an organ.

Cervical collar - An extra firm, contoured band of molded foam rubber or a similar synthetic material covered with stockinette; used to support neck injuries such as whiplash.

Cervical halter - A traction device prescribed for certain neck injuries or surgical procedures.

Cervix – The constricted portion of an organ or part; neck.

Cesarean section – An incision into the uterus through the abdominal wall to deliver a fetus.

CFC - Chlorofluorocarbon.

cg– Centigram.

Chafing - A reddened irritation of the skin caused by friction.

Chain of command – The organizational structure that traces responsibilities from the highest to lowest levels within a healthcare facility.

Chalazion – A small sebaceous cyst on the eyelid which appears as a bump and is caused by the inflammation of a blocked meibomian gland: a fat-secreting gland of the eyes. It differs from a stye (hordeolum) in that it is usually larger and is generally painless except for tenderness which occurs as it swells.

Challenge test pack – A device used in qualification, installation, and on-going quality assurance testing of hospital sterilizers.

Chamber (sterilizer) – An enclosed area of a sterilizer that holds products to be sterilized.

Change agent – A term that defines an individual or group who causes or accelerates change that is implemented by an organization.

Change management – The process of applying knowledge, tools, and resources to deal with change. It includes defining and implementing strategies, systems, procedures, communication, and technologies to navigate changes in external or internal conditions.

Change order – A revision to a construction purchase order issued by a buyer to a contractor or service provider.

Charge code – A code assigned to a specific item to assist in the reimbursement process.

Charge description master (CDM) – A comprehensive listing of items that could be billed to a patient, payer, or healthcare provider; also called charge master.

Charge system - A method of accounting for each item issued and charged to a patient or department.

Chelating agents - Chemicals that hold hard water minerals in solution and prevent soaps or detergents from reacting with the minerals.

Chemical indicators (CIs) - Systems that reveal a change in one or more predefined process parameters based on a chemical or physical change resulting from exposure to a process.

Chemical sterilization – A process using a chemical agent to render a product free of viable microorganisms.

Chemotherapy – The treatment of disease without injury to a patient with chemicals having a specific effect on microorganisms.

Chest stripper – An instrument used to remove tissue from rib bones.

Chest trocar - Thoracic trocar; a large-handled instrument with a sharp triangular tip used with a cannula to remove fluid from the chest cavity.

CHF – Congestive heart failure.

Chicken pox - Varicella; a rather mild, highly contagious viral disease characterized by fever and the appearance of vesicles (small fluid-filled blisters).

Chiropractor - A specialist who treats disease by manipulation of the spinal column.

Chisels - Wedge-shaped instruments used to cut or shape bone.

CHL - Certification in Healthcare Leadership; a certification program offered by the International Association of Healthcare Central Service Materiel Management (IAHCSMM).

Chloride – A compound commonly found in water that is created when chlorine is combined with another element or radical; examples are salt and hydrochloric acid.

Chlorofluorocarbon (CFC) – An inert (non-flammable) gas often mixed with a flammable gas to create an inflammable solution; has been used with ethylene oxide to create an inert gas.

Chlorophyll – A molecule in plants that absorbs sunlight and converts it to energy in a process called photosynthesis.

CHMMC - Certification in Healthcare Materiel Management Concepts; a certification program offered by the International Association of Healthcare Central Service Materiel Management (IAHCSMM)

Cholangiogram - The injection of a radiopaque dye to observe the common bile duct by means of x-rays.

Cholesterol - Organic, fat-like compound found in animal fat, bile blood, myelin, liver, and other parts of the body.

Chromium – A blue-white metallic element found naturally only in combination and used in alloys and electroplating.

Chromogenic - Producing a pigment.

Chromosome - Rod-shaped masses of chromatin (the genetic material that makes up DNA) that appear in the cell nucleus during mitosis. Chromosomes play an important part in cell division and transmit the cell's hereditary characteristics.

Chronic - Referring to a disease (illness) that is not severe but is continuous, recurring, protracted, and prolonged.

Chronic obstructive pulmonary disease (COPD) – A group of lung diseases that block airflow and make it increasingly difficult to breathe; examples are emphysema and chronic bronchitis.

Cidal – A word element that means having the power to kill such as bactericidal (will kill bacteria).

Cilia (sing; cilium) – Hair-like elements that spring from certain cells and, by their action, create currents in liquids. If the cells are fixed, the liquid is made to flow; if the cells are unicellular organisms suspended in the liquid, the cells move.

Circular electric bed - An electronically powered, circularly framed bed that promotes circulation in a bedridden patient by slow, continuous rotation of the body.

Circulating nurse - A surgical nurse who circulates in the operating room to monitor the procedure. The circulating nurse ensures that the conditions in the operating room remain safe and sterile. Circulating nurses also perform a wide variety of other tasks, such as helping to set up the operating room for surgery and documenting events during the procedure.

Circulation – The continuous movement of blood through the vessels of the body resulting from the pumping action of the heart.

Circumcision - Excision of the foreskin of the glans of the penis.

Circumduction - Circular movement at a joint.

Cirrhosis - Chronic disease, usually of the liver, in which active cells are replaced by inactive scar tissue.

CIS - Certified Instrument Specialist, a certification program offered by the International Association of Healthcare Central Service Materiel Management (IAHCSMM).

CJD – Creutzfeldt-Jakob Disease.

Clamp - A surgical device such as a hemostat used to compress blood vessels or tubing.

Class I medical devices (FDA) – These include low risk devices such as most hand-held surgical instruments and ultrasonic cleaners.

Class II medical devices (FDA) – These include most types of sterilization equipment and biological and chemical indicators.

Class III medical devices (FDA) – These are the most stringently regulated devices and include heart valves, pacemakers, and other life-sustaining devices.

Clean Air Act Amendments (1990) – A regulatory program administered by the federal Environmental Protection Agency to protect the earth's ozone layer; requires the use of chlorofluorocarbons in ethylene oxide sterilants.

Clean catch urine - A urine sample collected after the urethral opening and surrounding tissues have been cleansed.

Cleaning – The removal of all visible and non-visible soil and any other foreign material from medical devices being reprocessed.

Cleft lip - A congenital separation or division of the lip.

Clerk of Courts (or related title) – A person appointed by the court to work with the judge to oversee the management of case flow through the court system and to maintain court records.

Client/server relationship – The reliance of a less powerful computer (client) on another, more powerful computer (server) to receive services.

Climate survey (human resources) – A tool that solicits and assesses employee opinions, perceptions, and expectations about on-job factors including growth opportunities, management, working relationships, and the environment.

Clinical case - Pertaining to actual observation and treatment of a patient as a clinical or bedside case as opposed to a theoretical or experimental case.

Clip remover - An instrument used for the extraction or removal of metal clips from surgical wounds.

Clostridium - Genus of cylindrical-shaped bacteria which are anaerobic, gram-positive, and spore-forming.

cm – Centimeter.

CNS – Central nervous system.

CO – Carbon monoxide.

CO – Cardiac output.

CO_2 – Carbon dioxide.

CO_2 absorber -- A device used during the administration of anesthesia that contains an absorbent material such as soda lime to remove carbon dioxide from the gas exhaled by the patient.

Coaching – Positive reinforcement used by a manager to encourage employees to follow proper work practices and negative reinforcement to discourage employees from using improper work practices.

Coagulation - Clotting (as of blood).

Coccus - Round-shaped (spherical) bacteria.

Coccyx - Tail bone.

Cochlea – The coiled portion of the inner ear that contains the organs of hearing.

COLA – Cost of living adjustment.

Coliform (bacteria) – A group of intestinal microorganisms of which Escherichia coli is a member.

Collagen – A flexible white protein that gives strength and resilience to connective tissue including bone and cartilage.

Collar (cervical) - See cervical collar.

Colectomy - An operation to remove all or part of the colon. In a partial colectomy, the surgeon removes only the cancerous part of the colon and a small amount (called a margin) of surrounding healthy tissue.

Colonoscope - A thin tube-like medical device with a light and lens used to examine the inside of the entire colon and rectum that may include a tool used for tissue removal; inserted through the rectum into the colon.

Colony count – A determination of the number of visible clumps of bacteria derived from the multiplication of specific microorganisms on or in a culture medium.

Colony - Visible growth of microorganisms seen in culture medium; usually obtained from a single organism.

Colostomy - The surgical creation of an opening made at the surface of the abdomen to evacuate the bowels and to act as a substitute for the rectum and anus.

Colostomy appliance set - A ringed plastic bag, surgical adhesive, and an elastic waist belt used to cover the colostomy for fecal collection.

Colostomy belts - An elastic waistband that fits around a patient to hold the colostomy bag in place for fecal collection.

Colostomy irrigation - A kit containing a plastic irrigation bag and tubing, catheter, connector, and appliance collection bag for fecal material; used for irrigation to regulate the colostomy.

Colostomy pouch - A ringed, adhesive backed, plastic bag that fits over the stoma of the colostomy to collect fecal material.

Colposcope - An endoscopic instrument used in the examination of the cervix, vagina, or vulva; includes a magnifying lens used for the direct observation and study of the tissues of the cervix and vagina.

Colposcopy - A visual examination of the cervix and vagina using a colposcope to check for abnormalities; primarily performed to identify areas of cervical dysplasia in women with abnormal Pap smears; see colopscope.

Combining vowel – A letter, usually an "o," sometimes used to ease the pronunciation of a medical term.

Combustible – The ability to undergo a chemical process accompanied by the emission of heat, typically by combination with oxygen.

Combustible loading – The weight of combustible materials per square foot of area in which the materials are located.

Combustion – A chemical process accompanied by the rapid production of heat and light.

Commissioning (installation qualification) – The act of obtaining and documenting evidence that equipment has been provided and installed in accordance with its specifications, and that it functions within predetermined limits when operated in accordance with operating instructions.

Commode – A portable toilet.

Commode pan - A pail-like removable receptacle for a portable toilet.

Communicable – A disease whose causative agent is easily transmitted from person-to-person by direct or indirect contact.

Communicable disease - An illness that can be transmitted from one person to another directly or indirectly.

Communication – The process of transmitting information and understanding from one person to another by use of words and non-verbal expressions including body language.

Communication (formal) – Communication channels established by the healthcare organization that involve the official relationship of the persons sending and receiving the information.

Communication (informal) – Communication that flows through unofficial channels not directly connected with the healthcare organization and which is based upon unofficial (social) affiliation of members; see grapevine.

Comparison ratio (compensation) – A calculation made by dividing an employee's actual pay level by the mid-point of the employee's pay grade. A ratio greater than 1.0 indicates the employee's pay is above the salary range mid-point; a ratio less than 1.0 means the salary is below the range's mid-point; abbreviated "compa ratio."

Compensation – The total wages or salary including benefits paid to an employee.

Compensatory time-off – Compensation for overtime work that allows employees one and one-half hours of paid time-off in the future for each hour of overtime worked; also called "comp time."

Competency – A standard of knowledge, skills, and abilities that is required for successful job performance.

Competency checklist – A list of tasks used to monitor progress in a training program. Each task must be consistently performed in a way that meets quality and quantity output standards, and then it is marked as completed on the checklist; also called competency record.

Competency-based pay – A compensation system that recognizes employees who acquire a critical skill or knowledge; also called skill-based pay or knowledge-based pay.

Competitive bidding – A tactic used by purchasers who compare vendors' prices for products/services of equivalent quality to determine the least expensive price; also called competitive pricing.

Complaint (legal) – The first document filed with the Clerk of Courts by a person or entity claiming legal rights against another.

Complete blood count (CBC) - An analysis of blood undertaken with a group of hematological tests.

Compliance – The act of following identified regulations and standards.

Complication – A secondary illness imposed upon a person with a primary illness.

Compound – A substance composed of two or more chemical elements.

Compress - Material such as gauze or cloth folded and firmly pressed to a body part to prevent hemorrhage or moistened with water or medication to reduce inflammation or pain.

Compressed air - Air under greater-than-atmospheric pressure.

Compression - The act of squeezing together.

Compressor - A machine that compresses gases such as air.

Computed axial tomography (CAT or CT) – An imaging method in which multiple x-ray views taken from different angles are analyzed by computer to show a cross section of an area; used to detect tumors and other abnormalities; also called computerized tomography scan.

Concentration - The amount of a specified substance in a unit amount of another substance.

Condition of employment – Department or facility policies and work rules with which employees must comply. Example: Central Service employees must follow specific dress codes when working with bloodborne pathogens.

Conditional Accreditation (The Joint Commission) – Results when a health care organization was in Preliminary Denial of Accreditation, or the organization failed to resolve the requirements of a Provisional Accreditation; or it was not in substantial compliance with the applicable standards. The organization must remedy identified problem areas and subsequently undergo an on-site, follow-up survey.

Conditioning - Treatment of products within the sterilization cycle but before sterilant admission to attain a predetermined temperature and relative humidity; may be carried out at atmospheric pressure or under vacuum.

Condom - A rubber sheath designed to cover the penis during sexual intercourse to prevent infection or conception.

Condom drainage unit - A device used as an external catheter for males.

Conduction – A heat transfer method in which heat is absorbed by an item's exterior surface and passed inward to the next layer.

Conduction heating – A process in which heat is transmitted in a solid substance from molecule to molecule by molecular impact or agitation.

Conductivity (of water) - A measurement of the ability of water to carry an electrical current.

Confidentiality – The protection of specific patient and healthcare facility information.

Confidentiality (patient) – The right of a patient to have personal and identifiable medical information kept private.

Confidentiality agreement – A contract that restricts an employee or vendor from disclosing confidential information.

Conflict of interest – The situation that occurs when an employee has competing financial, professional, or personal interests that may interfere with his or her ability to adequately perform required duties without bias.

Congenital - Present at birth.

Congestive heart failure (CHF) - A condition in which the heart cannot pump enough blood to the body's other organs.

Conjunctiva – The membrane that lines the eyelid and covers the anterior part of the sclera.

Conjunctivitis - Inflammation of the conjunctiva of the eye.

Connecting tubing - Rubber or plastic tubing used to connect catheters and tubing to pump or drainage units.

Conscious sedation - An alternative to general anesthesia in patients for whom general anesthesia is refused or considered inadvisable that involves the administering of an anti-anxiety drug and an analgesic or local anesthetic.

Consignment (products) – Items that are available in a facility's inventory but which are owned by the manufacturer until used.

Consultant – An expert who contracts to assist organizations and/or their departments about specific issues.

Contagious - Highly communicable; easily transmitted.

Contaminate - To render unfit for use through introduction of a substance which is harmful or injurious.

Contaminated (linen) - Linen that has been soiled with blood or other potentially infectious materials.

Contaminated (sharps) - Any contaminated object that can penetrate the skin, including, but not limited to, needles, scalpels, broken glass, broken capillary tubes, and exposed ends of dental wires.

Contaminated (waste) - Potentially infectious materials disposed of by healthcare facilities such as soiled dressings, sharps, and fluids.

Contamination – The state of being soiled or infected by contact with infectious organisms or other material.

Continuous passive motion (CPM) device – A device that treats synovial joints (hip, knee, ankle, shoulder, elbow, wrist) following surgery or trauma including fracture and infection. The device moves the affected joint continuously without patient assistance.

Continuous quality improvement (CQI) – The scientific approach which applies statistical methods to improve work processes.

Contraception – The prevention of fertilization of an ovum or implantation of a fertilized ovum; birth control.

Contrast agent – A medium used by a radiologist in reading x-ray film that is administered to the patient before the x-ray procedure.

Control (management activity) – Coordinated steps to help Central Service leaders assure that actual operating results are on target with planned (budgeted) results.

Convalescence – The period during which recovery takes place following illness.

Convection (heating) – The transfer of heat in a fluid or gas from one place to another by the motion of the fluid or gas.

Conveyor – A transport system that moves products and materials over short distances; example: conveyor belt.

COPD – Chronic obstructive pulmonary disease

Copious - Present in a large amount such as a large volume of rinsing water.

Core (surgery work area) - The center of the surgery work area where items that may be quickly needed are often stored. Many cores have flash sterilizers for rapid instrument processing in emergencies.

Core values – Operating philosophies or principles that guide a facility's internal conduct and its relationships with external constituencies.

Cornea – The clear portion of sclera that covers the front of the eye.

Coronary - Referring to the heart or to the arteries supplying blood to the heart.

Coronary artery bypass (CAB) – A surgical procedure that re-routes the blood supply by bypassing blocked coronary arteries.

Coronary artery bypass graft (CABG) - A surgical procedure to restore the blood flow to the heart by bypassing clogged coronary arteries, usually with a saphenous vein graft taken from the leg.

Coronary artery disease (CAD) - A c ondition in which plaque builds up inside the coronary arteries; also called coronary heart disease.

Corrective action (financial management) – Tactics used to reduce negative variances between budgeted and actual costs; see negative variance.

Corrective action (human resources) – A written plan to resolve employee noncompliance with policies, procedures, or regulations; also the process of identifying steps to modify employee behaviors.

Corrosion – The act of wearing away gradually by a chemical reaction.

Corrosive - Having the power to corrode or wear away.

Cortex – The outer layer of an organ such as the brain, kidney, or adrenal gland.

Cosmetic surgery - A surgical procedure performed to improve the physical appearance of the body rather than for medical necessity.

Cost-benefit study – A financial analysis of the expected costs compared to the resulting benefits applicable to a specific project or activity. For example, a study may find that the cost of an instrument tracking system will be more than offset by reduced labor costs and the more consistent quality of processed instruments.

Cost containment – The control of inefficiencies in the consumption, allocation, or production of services that contribute to higher-than-necessary costs.

Cost of capital – The rate of return that an organization would receive if it invested its money elsewhere with similar risk.

Cost of living adjustment (COLA) – An annual compensation adjustment to offset a change in purchasing power as measured by the Consumer Price Index.

Cost trend – A record of costs incurred for a specific category of expense for several years or longer.

Cotton elastic bandage - A pressure dressing made of stretchable cotton fabric with interwoven strands of rubber.

Cotton-tipped applicators - Firmly wound tufts of cotton bonded to a stick used to cleanse or apply medications.

Coude catheter - Olive-tip catheter with a single drainage eye; used for male patients with urinary strictures.

Counseling – Actions or interactions that provide direction, guidance, or advice about an employee's decisions or courses of action.

Counter Stain – A second stain of a contrasting kind applied to a smear for the purpose of making the microorganisms treated with a primary stain more distinct.

CPR – Cardiopulmonary resuscitation.

CPT code – Current procedural terminology code.

CPU - Central processing unit.

CQI – Continuous quality improvement.

Cranial - Pertaining to the cranium.

Craniotomy - A medical term for all surgical procedures performed through an opening in the skull; examples include treating or removing cancer, clipping an aneurysm or removing a vascular malformation, and correcting a brain disorder or repairing a brain injury.

Cranium – The skull; the bony covering of the brain.

Crash cart - A set of trays on a wheeled cart used in hospital wards and emergency rooms that contains all the basic equipment needed to follow ACLS (Advanced Cardiac Life Support) and ALS (Advanced Life Support) protocols to potentially save a person's life; typically includes a defibrillator, intravenous medications such as epinephrine and atropine, and medical supplies such as latex gloves and alcohol swabs; also called a code cart.

Craze - Spider web cracking of plastics under chemical stress.

CRCST - Certified Registered Central Service Technician; a certification program offered by the International Association of Healthcare Central Service Materiel Management (IAHCSMM).

Creutzfeldt-Jakob disease (CJD) - A chronic brain-debilitating fatal disease; see prions.

Crisis – A change in a disease which indicates whether the result will be recovery or death.

Crisis management – The process of using pre-established guidelines to prepare for and respond to significant catastrophic events or incidents including fire, earthquake, severe storms, workplace violence, kidnapping, bomb threats, and terrorism in a safe and effective manner.

Critical items (Spaulding classification system) – Instruments or objects introduced directly into the bloodstream or other normally sterile body areas.

Critical parameters - Parameters that are essential to the sterilization process and that require monitoring.

Cross-contamination – Migration of contaminants from one person, object, or work location to another.

Cross-examine (legal) – The act of an attorney asking questions in court of a witness who has testified in a trial on behalf of the opposing party.

Cross-functional team – A group of employees from different departments within the healthcare facility that work together to resolve problems.

Cross-infection - Infection acquired from an animate or inanimate contaminated environment, usually accidentally.

Cross-training – A professional development activity that allows employees to learn how to perform tasks outside of their normal work responsibilities including those associated with a different job.

Crutch - An artificial support made of wood or metal to aid a patient unable to walk due to injury, disease, or other defects.

Crutch pad - A rubber pad used over the arm piece of a crutch to cushion the underarm.

Crutch tip – A rubber tip used on the bottom of a crutch to reduce slipping.

Cryosurgery - Treatment performed with an instrument that freezes and destroys abnormal tissues.

Cryotherapy - The use of low temperatures for medical therapy to a part of the body.

CSF – Cerebrospinal fluid.

C-suite – A term referring to those occupying the highest healthcare administrative positions. It is derived from the observation that the word "Chief" is frequently used in the position title. Example: Chief Financial Officer.

CSSD – Central sterile supply department.

CT – Computed axial tomography.

CT scan - Computed axial tomography scan.

CTS – Carpal tunnel syndrome.

cu - Cubic.

Culture (corporate) – The values and practices adopted by an organization that directly influence employee conduct and behavior; see organizational culture.

Culture (department) – The beliefs, values, and norms shared by department personnel that are considered valid and are passed on to new employees in the department.

Culture (microorganisms) - Growth of microorganisms on a nutrient medium; to grow microorganisms on such medium.

Culture medium – The substance or preparation used for the growth and cultivation of microorganisms.

Culture tube - A glass or plastic tubular container used to house microorganisms for growth.

Curbside in-services – Training programs generally offered in or near the work area that are flexible so staff members may attend at various times.

Current procedural terminology code (CPT code) - A numeric code assigned to every task or service that a medical practitioner may provide to a patient that is used by insurers to determine the amount of reimbursement a practitioner will receive.

Curet – See curette.

Curette - A scooped or spoon-shaped surgical instrument used for scraping dead tissue or growths from a body cavity.

Curettage – The removal of tissue or growths from a body cavity such as the uterus by scrapping with a curette.

Customer (internal) - Physicians, nurses, and other professional personnel served by Central Service personnel.

Customer service – The process of helping customers by addressing their needs in a timely manner.

Cutaneous - Referring to the skin.

Cutdown - A procedure creating an incision to reach a vein; used for passage of an intravenous catheter to administer intravenous (IV) fluids or transfusions.

CV - Cardiovascular.

CVA – Cerebrovascular accident.

CVP - Central venous pressure.

Cyanosis - Bluish color of the skin and mucous membranes resulting from insufficient oxygen in the blood.

Cyberspace – The world of information available through the internet.

Cycle (gravitation-displacement steam sterilization) - Sterilization cycle in which incoming steam displaces residual air through a port or drain in or near the bottom of the sterilizer chamber.

Cycle (sterilization) - Defined sequence of operational steps designed to achieve sterilization that is carried out in a sealed chamber.

Cycle buying - Purchasing method in which an order is placed at a scheduled interval.

Cycle time - Total elapsed time of a sterilization cycle from when the sterilizer door is closed and the cycle is activated until the cycle is completed and the door is opened.

Cystitis - Inflammation of the urinary bladder.

Cysto - Word element meaning bladder or cyst.

Cysto drape - Drape used to cover the area surrounding the genitalia for genito-urinary surgery.

Cystogram - Injection of a radiopaque dye into the bladder for an x-ray photograph.

Cystoscope - An endoscope fitted with a light that is designed to pass through the urethra to visually examine the bladder and ureters.

Cystoscopy - Visual inspection of interior of the bladder and examination of adjacent structures by means of a cystoscope introduced through the urethra.

Cytology – The study of cells.

Cytoplasm – The living matter of a cell between its membrane and nucleus.

D

D&C – Dilation or dilatation and curettage

D/W – Dextrose in water

Daily work records – A daily log of job tasks performed by individual employees over a specific time period; often used for benchmarking or job analysis activities.

Damage (legal) – The amount of money that the person initiating a lawsuit may be awarded.

Dashboard (department monitoring tool) – A collection of statistical data about a Central Service department's key performance indicators that indicates the extent to which goals are being attained; see key performance indicator.

Debridement - The removal of foreign material and devitalized or contaminated tissue from or adjacent to a traumatic or infected lesion until surrounding healthy tissue is exposed.

Decision (non-programmed) – A decision that requires a unique solution in an ill-structured situation in which the decision-maker has little or no experience.

Decision (programmed) – A decision made in a routine, well-structured situation that considers established rules, polices, and procedures and that incorporates experience and knowledge about what does and does not work in a specific situation.

Decontamination – Removing or reducing contamination by infectious organisms or other harmful substances.

Decontamination area – The location within a health care facility designated for collection, retention, and cleaning of soiled and/or contaminated items.

Decubitus ulcer – See bedsore.

Deep vein thrombosis (DVT) - A blood clot in one of the veins leading to the heart.

Defecation – The act of eliminating undigested waste from the digestive tract.

Defect – A variance from expected standards.

Defendant – A person against whom an action is brought in a court of law.

Defend-in-place – An emergency strategy in which occupants (patients) are relocated to a safe location on the same floor rather than being evacuated during an emergency.

Defibrillator - A device used to apply a brief electroshock to restore the rhythm of a defibrillating heart.

Deflocculate - To reduce or break-up into very fine particles.

Degeneration - Breaking down (as from age, injury, or disease).

Degerm - To remove bacteria and other microbes by mechanical cleaning and applying antiseptics or disinfectants.

Degree C - A reading on a Celsius or Centigrade temperature scale.

Degree F - A reading on a Fahrenheit temperature scale.

Dehydration - Excessive loss of body fluid.

Deionization – The process by which ions with an electrical charge are removed from water.

Deionize - To remove ions from (as water by ion exchange); demineralize.

Delegate – The process of assigning authority (power) to subordinates to do work that a manager at a higher organizational level would otherwise do.

Delivery invoice – A document signed by an authorized representative of the healthcare facility when items are delivered to transfer ownership to the facility. The delivery invoice is the source of vendor charges to the facility.

Demagnetizer – Device used to remove a magnetic field from instruments, usually needle holders.

Democratic (leadership style) – A leadership approach in which staff members are encouraged to participate in the decision-making process.

Demotion – A permanent reassignment to a position with a lower pay grade, skill requirement, or responsibility level than the employee's current position.

Denatured alcohol - Alcohol that has been rendered unfit for use as a beverage by the addition of substances which impart an unpleasant odor and taste; examples include wood alcohol and benzene.

Denial of Accreditation (The Joint Commission) – Results when a health care organization has been denied accreditation and all review and appeal opportunities have been exhausted.

Density – The degree of compactness; closely set or thickness.

Deoxyribonucleic acid (DNA) - One of two nucleic acids; essential for biological inheritance.

Depigmentation - Loss of skin color.

Deposition (legal) – The activity of taking and recording a witness's testimony under oath in a place away from the courtroom before trial.

Depreciation – The process to determine the value of a fixed asset during a specific accounting period that is assumed to be "used up" during the period.

Dermatitis - Inflammation of the skin.

Dermatome - A surgical instrument used to produce thin slices of skin from a donor area to use them for making skin grafts.

Dermis - True skin; the deeper part of the skin.

Designer – An unlicensed person who typically plans changes that do not relate to regulatory (building code) requirements.

Detergent – A cleaning agent composed of a "surface wetting agent" which reduces surface tension, a "builder" which is the principle cleaning agent, and a "sequestering" or "chelating agent" to suspend the soil; detergents may also have additional additives such as blood solvents or rust inhibitors; any chemical which causes oil or grease to dissolve in water and cleans the item on which it is used. Unlike soap, detergents do not contain fats and lye.

Detergent/germicide – A combination of a cleaning agent and a disinfectant.

Detergent/sanitizer – A combination of chemicals which possess antibacterial and cleaning properties.

Dextrose - Glucose; simple sugar.

Dextrose 10 percent saline - An intravenous solution used as a calorie and salt supplement.

Dextrose 20 percent water - An intravenous solution, diuretic in action, that may be used to reduce edema.

Dextrose 5 percent 0.25 saline - An intravenous solution used for fluid replacement in dehydrated patients.

Dextrose 5 percent 0.33 sodium chloride - An intravenous solution used to open a vein before administering whole blood.

Dextrose 5 percent lactated Ringer's solution - An intravenous solution used for fluid and electrolyte replacement.

Dextrose 5 percent saline solution - An intravenous solution used for fluid and body salt replacement.

Dextrose 5 percent water - An intravenous solution used as a source of calories and water.

DHS – Dynamic hip screw.

Diabetes mellitus - Disease in which glucose is not oxidized in body tissues for energy because of insufficient insulin.

Diagnosis – The identification of an illness.

Diagnostic related groups (DRGs) – A system developed for Medicare as part of the prospective payment system to classify hospital cases into groups that are expected to require similar facility resources.

Dialysis – A method to separate molecules in solution based on differences in their rates of diffusion through a semi-permeable membrane; method for removing nitrogen waste products from the body by hemodialysis or peritoneal dialysis.

Diaphragm – The dome-shaped muscle under the lungs that flattens during inhalation; a separating membrane or structure.

Diarrhea - Loose and frequent bowel movements.

Diathermy - One of the two types of electrocautery. With this type, the active and receiving electrodes are both placed at the site of cauterization. The probe is usually in the shape of a forceps with each tine forming one electrode, and only the tissue between the electrodes is cauterized; also called bipolar electrocautery.

DIC – Disseminated intravascular coagulation.

DIFF, diff – Differential blood count.

Differential blood count (DIFF, diff) – A measure of the percentage of each type of white blood cell in the blood and whether there are any abnormal or immature cells.

Differential staining - Staining techniques to distinguish between different bacteria.

Diffusion – The movement of molecules from a region of higher concentration to a region of lower concentration.

Digestion - The process of breaking down food into absorbable particles.

Digital subtraction angiography (DSA) – A method of taking images of arteries, veins, and organs of the body using complex computerized x-ray equipment.

Dilation and curettage (D&C) – A minor operation in which the cervix is expanded enough (dilation) to permit the cervical canal and uterine lining to be scraped with a spoon-shaped instrument called a curette (curettage). This procedure also is called D and C.

Dilation - Widening of a part such as the pupil of the eye, blood vessel, or uterine cervix.

Dilator - An instrument or drug that expands an organ or body part.

Diphtheria – An acute, infectious disease of the mucous membranes of the upper respiratory tract characterized by patches of pseudomembrane and caused by Corynebacterium diphtheriae.

Diplococcus - Pairs of cocci.

Direct contact – The spread of disease directly from person-to-person.

Direct impact (The Joint Commission) – A requirement for which noncompliance is likely to create an immediate risk to patient safety or the quality of care being provided.

Disaster (external) – A situation in which activities external to the facility affect departmental or facility operations.

Disaster (internal) – A situation with the potential to cause harm or injury to CSSD or other employees, or where the loss of utilities may drastically impact department operations.

Discharge (involuntary employment termination) – The termination of an employee based on disciplinary actions or for violating a major work rule or policy.

Disciplinary action – The oral and/or written process of reprimanding employees who do not follow performance standards or policies.

Discovery phase (legal action) – The time during which a party to a lawsuit and applicable attorneys obtain all possible information about the lawsuit before the trial actually begins.

Discovery process (legal action) – The process by which eligible, non-privileged information relevant to either party's claim or defense is provided to the other party before a trial begins.

Discrimination – Unequal treatment of persons for reasons that do not relate to their legal rights or abilities. Federal and state laws prohibit discrimination in employment, housing, pay rates, promotion rights, educational opportunities, civil rights, and use of facilities based on race, nationality, creed, color, age, sex, or sexual orientation.

Discrimination (workplace) – Unfavorable or unfair treatment on the basis of an individual's race, religion, gender, national origin, disability, age and, in some states and communities, sexual orientation.

Disease – A state of illness characterized by marked symptoms caused by an infectious agent producing a definite pathological pattern.

Disinfectant – A chemical which kills most pathogenic organisms but not spores; is not a sterilant.

Disinfectant/detergent – A chemical compound that contains both detergent and disinfectant; usually the action of both is compromised because of the combination.

Disinfection - Destruction of nearly all pathogenic microorganisms on an inanimate surface.

Disinfestation - Destruction of insects, rodents, or other animals which transmit infections to other animals, humans, or their surroundings.

Dismiss (legal) – A ruling by the judge that all or part of the plaintiff's lawsuit should be terminated.

Displacement – An ionic change in which one element exchanges with another element by oxidation or reduction; a chemical change in which one element, molecule, or radical is removed by another.

Disposable - An item or product designed to be used only once and discarded.

Dissection - The process of disassembling and observing something to determine its internal structure. In medical pathology, dissection refers to a tear in the wall of a blood vessel. The term also applies to the separation of the layers of arterial tissue in the aorta as a result of blood being forced out into the wall of the aorta through a tear in the innermost layer of tissue. See also: tissue dissection.

Disseminated intravascular coagulation (DIC) – A serious disorder in which the proteins that control blood clotting become abnormally active.

Dissociation - Physical breaking apart of a molecule.

Distal - Farther from the origin of a structure or from a given reference point.

Distill - To vaporize by heat, and condensing and collecting the volatilized product.

Distillation – The process of changing from liquid to vapor to liquid; a process for removing impurities from liquids.

Distilled water - Water that has been heated to its boiling point, vaporized, cooled, and condensed into liquid form; a condensate with no minerals and a pH of 7.0.

Distribution – The movement of (primarily consumable) supplies throughout the facility from the storeroom to clinical units and reprocessed supplies from Central Service to the operating room.

Distributor – An intermediary who sells specific (branded) products within a specifically-defined sales territory.

Diversity – The concept that people are unique with individual differences stemming from race, ethnicity, gender, socio-economic status, age, and physical abilities, among others.

dl – deciliter (100 ml).

DM – Diabetes mellitus.

DME - Durable medical equipment.

DNA – Deoxyribonucleic acid.

DNR – Do not resuscitate.

DO – Doctor of Osteopathy.

Doctor's (Physician's) preference card – A document that identifies a specific physician's needs (requests and preferences) for instruments, equipment, supplies, and utensils for a specific procedure.

Dominant (gene) - Referring to a gene that is always expressed if present.

DON – Director of Nursing.

Don – Donor.

Dorsalis pedis – The dorsal artery of the foot.

Dorsal - Toward the back; posterior.

Dosimeter – A device that measures the amount of a hazardous substance such as EtO or hydrogen peroxide (H_2O_2) to which a person has been exposed.

Douche - A stream of water or vapor directed against a body part or cavity for cleansing and medical applications.

Down time rate (equipment) – Number of down days/ Number of devices (x) 365.

Downsize – The process of reducing the workforce size by actions including the elimination of positions and/or management layers and through job restructuring.

DPT – Diphtheria, Pertussis, and Tenanus (toxoids/ vaccine).

Dr – Doctor.

Drain - A tube inserted into the opening of a wound or cavity to promote discharge of fluids.

Drainage bag - A plastic bag with connecting tubing used to collect fluid from patients with in-dwelling drains.

Drape – A woven or non-woven protective cloth used to maintain sterility.

DRG – Diagnostic-related groups.

Dressing - A bandage or covering for an external wound.

Droplet infection – An infection transmitted by small drops (particles) of sputum or nasal discharges expelled into the air while talking, coughing, or sneezing.

Dry-heat sterilizer – A hot-air sterilizer; an oven-like apparatus powered by electricity to sterilize items by subjecting them to high temperatures for long exposure periods.

DSA – Digital subtraction angiography.

Duct – A tube or vessel.

Due diligence – The process of conducting an investigation and analysis to determine the details of a specific issue before making a decision.

Duodenum – The first portion of the small intestine.

Durable medical equipment (DME) – Medical equipment items such as walkers, wheelchairs, or hospital beds that are placed in a patient's home to facilitate treatment and/ or rehabilitation.

Dust cover – A protective plastic bag used to maintain the sterility of an item by protecting it from the environment; also called sterility maintenance cover.

D-value – The amount of time required to kill 90% of the microorganisms present.

DX, Dx, dx – Diagnosis.

Dye – A coloring material used for staining or coloring bacteria for microscopic examination.

Dynamic hip screw – A screw used for internal fixation of fractures of the hip and parts of the thigh.

Dysentery - Inflamed condition of intestines accompanied by pain and diarrhea.

Dysfunction – An impaired or abnormal function.

Dyspnea - Difficult or labored breathing.

E

EAP – Employee assistance program.

Ear syringe - A ringed syringe used for irrigation of the ear.

Ebonize - Exposure of an instrument to a chemical dip which blackens the metal.

ECF – Extracellular fluid.

EKG – Electrocardiogram.

Echocardiogram - A medical test in which sound waves are used to produce an image of the heart through a non-invasive procedure.

E-commerce – The process of conducting business and sharing information by using the computer and telecommunication networks including the internet.

Economic order quantity (purchasing system) – A purchasing system that uses mathematical calculations to determine purchase quantities that yield the lowest total variable costs.

ECT – Electroconvulsive therapy.

Ectopic pregnancy - A pregnancy in which the fertilized ovum is implanted outside the uterus.

Ectoplasm – The outer clear zone of the cytoplasm of a one-celled organism.

ED – Emergency Department.

Edema – The presence of abnormally large amounts of fluid in intercellular tissue spaces of the body.

EDI - Electronic data interchange.

EEG – Electroencephalogram.

EEOC – Equal Employment Opportunity Commission.

Effect analysis – A tactic to study the consequences of identified failures; see failure mode and effect analysis.

Effecter - An organ or cell that carries out a response to a nerve impulse.

Effusion – The escape of fluid into a space or part; the fluid itself.

Ejaculation – The expulsion of semen through the urethra.

Ejaculatory duct – The duct formed by the joining of the seminal vesicles with the vas deferens, through which semen moves during ejaculation.

EL – Excursion limit.

Elastic bandage - A flexible, stretchable fabric made with interwoven strands of rubber used as a pressure dressing.

Electrodes - Mediums used between an electric conductor and the object to which the current is to be applied. In electrotherapy, electrodes are instruments with a point or surface from which to transmit electric current to the body of a patient or to another instrument; in electrodiagnosis, they are needles or metal plates used to stimulate or record the electrical activity of tissue.

Electrocardiogram (ECG) - The tracing or recording of the electric impulses of the heart.

Electrocardiograph (ECG or EKG) – An instrument to study the electric activity of the heart; the record made is an electrocardiogram.

Electrocautery - The process of destroying tissue with electricity; frequently used to stop bleeding of small vessels or for cutting through soft tissue such as abdominal fat in a laparotomy or breast tissue in a mastectomy.

Electrocoagulation - Electrosurgical procedures used to treat hemorrhage and to ablate (remove) tumors, mucosal lesions, and refractory arrhythmias.

Electroconvulsive therapy (ECT) – A procedure that uses electric currents passed through the brain to cause a brief seizure.

Electroencephalogram (EEG) - The tracing of recordings of the electric impulses of the brain.

Electroencephalograph (EEG) – An instrument used to study electric activity of the brain; record made is an electroencephalogram.

Electrolyte – A compound that forms ions in solution; a substance that conducts an electric current in solution.

Electron irradiation – A procedure used by some manufacturers for commercial sterilization.

Electromyogram (EMG) – A test used to record the electrical activity of muscles.

Electron – A negatively-charged particle that moves around the nucleus (central core) of an atom.

Electronic data interchange (EDI) – The automated exchange of data and documents in a standardized format. A common use is the exchange of routine business transactions between computers in a standard format using standard communication protocols; example: an electronic order placed by a facility's purchasing department to a vendor.

Electronic requisition – A request for equipment, products, or other items made electronically by users to those responsible for the items requested.

Electronic thermometer - An electric device with disposable probe used to take oral and rectal temperatures.

Electroplating - To plate with an adherent continuous coating by electrodeposition.

Electrostatic - Pertaining to the attractions and repulsions of electrical charges.

Electrosurgical generator - Medical equipment used during electrosurgery with a handpiece including one or several electrodes; also called power supply or waveform generator.

Element - One substance from which all matter is made; a substance that cannot be decomposed into a simpler substance.

Elements of performance (The Joint Commission) – Specific performance expectations that must be in place for an organization to provide safe, high quality care, treatment, and services.

Embolus – A blood clot or other obstruction in the circulation system; the condition is an embolism.

Embryo - Developing offspring during the first two months of pregnancy.

Emergency – An unexpected illness or injury that requires immediate medical care.

Emergency Medical Treatment and Labor Act (EMTALA) – A federal act that requires hospitals to provide emergency treatment to individuals regardless of their insurance status or ability to pay.

Emergency room (ER) – An area in which patients are received, evaluated, and treated; usually involves treatment for disease or injury that cannot wait for a visit to a doctor's office; also called emergency department (ED).

Emerson suction pump - A three-bottle suction unit with a variety of pressures used for thoracic suction.

Emesis -Vomiting.

Emesis Basin - A shallow basin with a kidney-shaped footprint and sloping walls; also called kidney basin.

EMG – Electromyogram.

Emotional intelligence – A type of social ability that allows persons to monitor their and others' emotions, to discriminate among them, and to use the information to guide their own thinking and behavior.

Emphysema – A pulmonary disease characterized by dilation and alveoli destruction.

Employee assistance program (EAP) -- An employer-provided intervention to identify and help employees resolve marital, financial, emotional, family, substance/alcohol abuse, or other personal problems that may adversely affect their job performance.

Employee benefits – Non-wage or salary compensation paid to employees including sick leave, vacation pay, retirement contributions, and medical and dental insurance; also called fringe benefits.

Employee engagement – The process of creating a work environment that empowers employees to make discretionary decisions that affect their jobs.

Employee group (formal) – A group of employees identified by the facility's organization chart.

Employee group (informal) – A group of employees from the same or different work groups who form an unofficial group of staff members.

Employee handbook – A permanent reference guide for employers and employees that contains information about the healthcare facility, its goals, and its current employment policies and procedures.

Empowerment – The act of granting authority to employees to make key decisions within their areas of responsibility.

Empyema – The accumulation of pus in a body cavity, especially the chest.

Emulsification – The dispersion of two mutually immiscible (unable to be mixed) liquids.

Emulsify - To break down large volumes of fats, oils, and greases into small globules which are held in suspension.

Emulsion - A mixture of two liquids not mutually soluble; the process for breaking up oils and fats into small particles which are held in suspension and making it easier to clean items.

Encephalitis - Inflammation of the brain.

Encephalogram - The injection of air into the cerebrospinal canal to allow for an x-ray of the brain.

Encephalomyelitis - Inflammation of the brain and spinal cord.

Encumbrance (accounting) - The process of identifying the amount of budgeted money remaining for Central Service department expenses as the budget year evolves.

End of life (instruments) – Term to describe used instrumentation that has worn to the point it cannot be repaired or refurbished.

End user – The healthcare facility; the buyer of a product.

Endemic disease - One that occurs more or less continuously throughout a community.

Endocardial - Pertaining to or within the heart.

Endocarditis - Inflammation of the endocardium (lining membrane) of the heart including heart valves.

Endocardium – The membrane that lines the heart chambers and covers the valves.

Endocrine – A gland that secretes directly into the bloodstream.

Endogenous - Originating within the organism.

Endometrium – The lining of the uterus.

Endoscope - A rigid or flexible device consisting of a tube with a light and a lens on the end which may be inserted into a body opening or incision; typically used to examine hollow organs inside the body including the esophagus, stomach, duodenum, colon, or rectum, but also used to take tissue from the body for testing. Endoscopes can be attached to a camera to take color photographs of the inside of the body or for viewing on a video screen.

Endoscopy - A procedure used to examine, biopsy, or surgically treat a variety of conditions. Types of endoscopy include arthroscopy (joints), bronchoscopy (bronchial tubes and lungs), colonoscopy/sigmoidoscopy (large intestine), colposcopy (vagina, cervix), gastroscopy (stomach and small intestine), laparoscopy (abdomen), and others.

Endothelium - Epithelium that lines the heart, blood vessels, and lymphatic vessels.

Endotoxin – A toxin (poison) confined inside a microorganism that is only released when the microorganism is broken down or dies.

Endotracheal - Pertaining to or within the trachea.

Enema - Injection of fluid into the rectum for cleansing.

Engineering controls - Controls such as sharps disposal containers and self-sheathing needles that isolate or remove bloodborne pathogen hazards from the workplace.

ENT – Ear, nose, and throat.

Enteral Nutrition (infusion) pump – A device that provides nutrition to patients who cannot ingest food because of recent surgery or because various digestive organs do not function properly; also called feeding pump.

Enteric bacteria - Bacteria living in or isolated from the intestinal tract.

Enteric - Pertaining to the intestines.

Entrained - Trapped in the stream; example: water can be trapped in the stream of steam.

Environment – The space that surrounds or encompasses a person or an object.

Environmental impact study – A study that considers safety concerns applicable to the environment, employees, and community.

Environmental Protection Agency (EPA) – Creates and enforces laws relating to cleaner water, air, and land. Two major acts that affect Central Service are The Federal Insecticide, Fungicide, and Rodenticide Act (FIFRA), and the 1990 Clean Air Acts Amendments.

Enzymatic solution – A solution containing special enzymes that dissolve proteinaceous materials.

Enzyme – A substance that initiates chemical changes such as fermentation without participating in them; a catalyst, usually protein, produced by a living cell with a specific action and optimum activity at a definite pH value.

EO (EtO) – Ethylene Oxide.

EPA - Environmental Protection Agency.

Epicardium – The membrane that forms the outermost layer of the heart wall.

Epidemic (disease) - An outbreak of sudden rapid spread and growth of an infectious disease.

Epidemiologist - A specialist in epidemic diseases.

Epidemiology – The study of the occurrence and distribution of disease; usually refers to epidemics.

Epidermis – The outermost layer of the skin.

Epididymus – The tube that carries sperm cells from the testes to the vas deferens.

Epiglottis - Leaf-shaped cartilage that covers the larynx during swallowing.

Epistaxis - To bleed from the nose.

Epithelium - The cells that line hollow organs and glands and those that make up the body's outer surface.

Equal Employment Opportunity Commission (EEOC) – A federal government agency that enforces provisions of Title VII of the Civil Rights Act of 1964.

Equipment (capital) - Relatively expensive assets such as sterilizers or washers that require significant advance planning for their purchase.

Equipment utilization rate - Days used ÷ Number of devices (x) 365.

ER – Emergency Room

ERA – Estrodiol receptor assay

ERCP (endoscopic retrograde cholangiopancreatography) - A procedure to x-ray the common bile duct.

ERS – Event-related sterility

Ergonomics – The process of changing work or working conditions to reduce employee fatigue or discomfort.

Erythema - Redness of the skin.

Erythrocyte - Red blood cell (corpuscle).

Erythrocyte sedimentation rate (ESR) - A test that indirectly measures how much inflammation is in the body.

ESC - Evidence of Standards Compliance (The Joint Commission).

Esophageoscope - An endoscope used to visually examine the esophagus.

Esophagus – A tube that carries food from the throat to the stomach.

ESR – Erythrocyte sedimentation rate

Estrogen – A group of female sex hormones that promotes development of the uterine lining and maintain secondary sex characteristics.

Ethics – Written and/or unwritten standards about appropriate and inappropriate moral conduct or behavior by an individual or an organization.

Ethics (medical) – Application of codes of ethics or guidelines adopted for the protection of patients, families and the healthcare facility.

Ethylene oxide (EO or EtO) – A gas used in low temperature sterilization; performs as a very effective general purpose sterilant for items that are heat or moisture-sensitive; also used as a fumigant.

Ethylene oxide sterilizer - A sterilizer with a locked chamber and humidity control used to sterilize instruments, supplies, and other items that cannot withstand high heat or humidity.

Etiology – The study of the cause of a disease or the theory of its origin.

EtO (EO)- Ethylene oxide.

Eustachian tube – The tube that connects the middle ear cavity to the throat; auditory tube.

Evacuation (body cavity) - The act of vacating or emptying a body cavity.

Evacuation (emergency) – The act of removing people from an area such as evacuating staff and patients from a hospital in a fire.

Event-related shelf life – The concept that a package is considered sterile until some event makes it unsterile (contaminated).

Evidence of Standards Compliance (ESC; The Joint Commission) – An electronic, extranet-based report submitted by a surveyed organization in response to Requirements for Improvement ("Not Compliant" standards) that are identified as the result of The Joint Commission survey. This report details the actions at the Element of Performance level taken by the organization to comply with the standards or to clarify why it believes it was in compliance with the standards at the time of survey.

Ex – Examination.

Exacerbation – An increase in the severity of a disease.

Exam gloves - Disposable gloves made from a latex-free material or vinyl worn for protection during patient contact.

Exc – Excision.

Exchange cart system – An inventory system in which desired inventory items are placed on a cart assigned a specific location. A second, duplicate cart is maintained in another location, and the two carts are exchanged once daily to ensure that sufficient supplies are always available.

Excrete - To eliminate or separate waste matter from an organism.

Excretion - To eliminate or give off waste products such as feces, perspiration, or urine.

Excursion limit (EL) - A certain amount of hazardous substance beyond which a person should not be exposed to in a specified period. Example: the EtO EL is 5 ppm in 15 minutes.

Exempt employees – Salaried employees who meet a Fair Labor Standards Act (FLSA) exemption test and are not entitled to overtime pay.

Exfoliate - To come off in strips or sheets; particularly the stripping of the skin after certain exanthematous (rash) diseases.

Exit interview – An interview used to identify factors prompting an employee to resign.

Exotoxin – A soluble poisonous substance excreted by a living microorganism; can be obtained in bacteria-free filtrates without death or disintegration of the microorganism.

Expedite (purchasing) – Facilitating the delivery of products previously ordered or compliance with contracts for services that have been negotiated with suppliers.

Expense – Any cost incurred to provide the processed products and services provided by the Central Service department.

Expiration date – The date calculated by adding a specific period of time to the date of manufacture or sterilization of a medical device or component that defines its estimated useful life.

Expiration statement – A statement indicating that the contents of a package are sterile indefinitely unless the integrity of the package is compromised.

Exposure (employee) – The chance for an employee to be affected during the course of working in Central Service through any route of entry: inhalation, ingestion, skin contact, or absorption.

Exposure incident - A specific eye, mouth, other mucous membrane, or non-intact skin contact with blood, or other potentially infectious materials that results from the performance of an employee's duties.

Exposure time – The time for which the sterilizer's chamber is maintained within the specified range for temperature, sterilant concentration, pressure, and humidity.

EXT – External.

Extended cycles – Sterilization cycles that fall outside of the traditional cycles used in the Central Service department because exposure times exceed standard steam sterilization times.

External construction – Renovation and/or new construction that involves the outside of a healthcare facility.

External solutions - Solutions normally used for irrigating, topical application, and surgical use given orally or by inhalation.

Extracellular - Outside the cell.

Extracellular fluid – Body fluid that is not contained in the cell.

Extraction – The use of physical force (usually centrifugal or strike/impact) to remove excess water from a wash load prior to drying.

Extraneous - Outside the organism and not belonging to it.

Extrinsic - From without.

Exudate - Accumulation of a fluid in a cavity or matter that penetrates through the vessel walls into adjoining tissue.

Eye mask - A covering used to keep dressing in position following eye or cataract surgery.

Eye pad - An oval gauze dressing used on the eye to absorb drainage.

Eye shield - A device used to cover and protect the eye.

F

F – Fahrenheit

F – Female

Facultative - Having the power to do something but not ordinarily doing it; capable of adapting to different conditions; example: a facultative anaerobe (microorganism) can live in the presence of oxygen but does not ordinarily do so.

Fahrenheit – The thermometer scale in which the space between the freezing point and the boiling point of water is 180°; 32° is the freezing point and 212° is the boiling point. To convert from Fahrenheit to Centigrade: $5/9 \, (°F - 32) = °C$.

Failure mode – An element in failure mode and effect analysis, a process improvement technique that recognizes errors can potentially occur during any given process; see failure mode and effect analysis.

Failure mode and effect analysis (FMEA) – A process to predict the adverse outcomes of various human and machine failures to prevent future adverse outcomes.

Fair Labor Standards Act (FLSA) – Laws administered by the U.S. Department of Labor that address compensation and child labor concerns.

Fallopian tubes - Slender tubes that convey the ova (eggs) from the ovaries to the uterus.

Families (chemicals) - Groups of chemicals that have similar characteristics.

Fascia – A band or sheet of fibrous connective tissue.

Fasting blood sugar (FBS) – A test that measures blood glucose after one has not eaten for eight hours.

FBS – Fasting blood sugar

FCS - Fellowship in Central Service; a certification program offered by the International Association of Healthcare Central Service Materiel Management (IAHCSMM).

FDA – Food and Drug Administration.

Feasibility study – The examination of a proposed plan or project to determine whether it can be successfully implemented.

Febrile - Characterized by or pertaining to fever.

Feces - Waste material discharged from the large intestine; excrement; stool.

Federal Insecticide, Fungicide, and Rodenticide Act (FIFRA) – Regulations administered by the Environmental Protection Agency that address the safety and effectiveness of all anti-microbial products including disinfectants and sanitizers.

Feedback – A step in communication that occurs when the listener asks a question, repeats information, or otherwise helps the speaker to know if the message has been correctly received.

Feedback (to question) – The response given to a question or a broader-scale request for information.

Feeding tube - A nasogastric tube used as a pathway to the stomach for the feeding of liquids and semi-solid foods.

Felt - A fabric of matted and compressed fibers used as padding for orthopedic procedures.

Fem – Femur.

Femoral - Pertaining to the femur or thigh bone.

Femur (Fem) - Upper leg bone.

Fenestrated - Having openings.

Fermentation - Decomposition of complex organic molecules under the influence of ferments or enzymes; usually associated with living microorganisms.

Fertilization – The union of an ovum and a spermatozoan.

Fetal - Pertaining to a fetus.

Fetus - Developing offspring from the third month of pregnancy until birth.

Fever - Abnormally high body temperature.

Fever of undetermined origin (FUO) – An unexplained fever.

Fiberoptic - A bundle of thread-like flexible, transparent fibers used in an instrument to transmit light and images such as for viewing body cavities.

Fiber optic bronchoscopy (FOB) – A procedure that allows a clinician to examine the breathing passages of the lungs.

Fibrin - Blood protein that forms a blood clot.

Fibula – A smaller bone of the lower leg.

FIFO – see First in, first out.

FIFRA - Federal Insecticide, Fungicide, and Rodenticide Act (FIFRA).

File – A block of information containing a program, document, or collection of data. Example: a text file contains lines of information that can be sent to a computer or printer with ordinary operating system commands.

Filiform - Thread-shaped dilators; used to dilate narrow ureteral strictures.

Filter (rigid container system) – A device secured to a rigid sterilization container's lid and/or bottom that allows passage of air and sterilants but provides a microbial barrier.

Filter retention system (rigid container system) – A mechanism on a rigid sterilization container that secures disposable filters in place.

Filtrate – A liquid that has passed through a filter.

Fimbriae - Finger-like projections extending from the fallopian tubes that draw ova (eggs) into the fallopian tube.

Financial statements – Documents that detail an organization's financial position.

Finger cot - A small rubber shield placed over a finger for protection against soiling of infectious materials.

Fire rating – A standard measured in the time (minutes or hours) that a product such as a door can withstand exposure to fire test conditions.

Firewall – A network link through which only authorized data can pass that keeps computers safe from hackers and hardware failures that occur elsewhere.

First in, first out (FIFO) – A stock rotation system in which the oldest product (that which has been in storage the longest) is used first.

Fiscal year – The twelve-month period that is the facility's and Central Service department's budget year.

Fissure – A deep groove.

Fitness for duty – Written information from a licensed medical practitioner used by an employer to determine a person's ability to perform specific job functions. This information is required to enable employees to resume full or modified duties after time-off due to illness or injury.

Fixed assets – Things of value that are not consumed during normal operations in the Central Service department; examples are equipment, building or space, and facility improvements.

Fixed costs – Costs that do not change in relation to the volume of processing output in the Central Service department; examples are salaried labor and negotiated service contracts.

Flagella - Long, hair-like processes extending from the cell wall of a microorganism that helps an organism to move (especially in liquids).

Flammable – A combustible substance that ignites very easily, burns intensely, or has a rapid rate of flame spread.

Flash point – The lowest temperature at which the vapor of a combustible liquid can be ignited in the air.

Flash sterilization – The process by which unwrapped instruments are sterilized for immediate use when an emergency situation arises; process of sterilizing an item that is not packaged.

Flash sterilizer – A sterilizer that uses higher temperatures for shorter exposure times for emergency sterilization of dropped instruments.

Flat fee (instrument repair pricing) – A financial arrangement in which a repair vendor charges a pre-established fee for all instrument repair services performed for a facility during a specified time period.

Flatus - Gas in the digestive tract.

Flexion – A bending motion that decreases the angle between bones at a joint.

Flex time – A work schedule comprised of variable work hours and start times that is agreed to by the employer and employee. Flex time employees in healthcare positions typically work during peak volume and short-staff times.

Flora - Plant life; more specifically, plants adapted for living in a specific environment or period.

Flow chart – A graphic representation of the stages in a process or system or the steps required to solve a problem.

Flow meter – A device used to measure the flow of fluids or the air to measure respiration.

Fluff – A post-operative dressing; loosely woven and folded gauze.

Fluid invasion - Damage to powered surgical instruments when water or solution enters the instrument's internal components.

Fluoroscopy - An x-ray machine capable of producing both still images and "real-time" motion of the joints or vertebrae; often used to visualize intervertebral joint motion through flexion and extension of the neck or back or to place a syringe needle at a targeted site.

FOB - Fiber optic bronchoscopy.

Focal infection – A localized site of more or less chronic infection from which bacteria or their by-products are spread to other parts of the body.

Foley catheter - A double lumen rubber or plastic indwelling urethral catheter with a balloon which, when inflated, holds the catheter within the bladder.

Foley catheter plug - A stopper used to plug the lumen of a Foley catheter.

Fomite – An inanimate object that can transmit bacteria.

Food and Drug Administration (FDA) – A federal regulatory agency that ensures foods, cosmetics, human and veterinary drugs, biological products, medical devices, and electronic products emitting radiation are safe and effective; administers pre- and post-market medical device requirements, MedWatch, medical device classifications, and medical device recalls.

Foot candle – The amount of light equivalent to that produced by one standard candle at a distance of one foot.

Foot pump – A device that artificially stimulates the venous plantar plexus (the large vein located in the foot); increases blood circulation in bed-ridden patients by simulating the motion of blood produced during walking.

Footboard - A device placed at the foot of a bed to support the proper alignment of the foot; used to prevent foot drop.

Forceps – An instrument for grasping, holding firmly, or exerting traction upon objects.

Forging (instrument manufacture) – To form by heating and hammering.

Formaldehyde – A class of disinfectants most often used to disinfect hemodialysis equipment; also used as a preservative and fumigant. Use with caution because of its potential carcinogenic effect and irritating fumes.

Fox postnasal balloon - A device with an inflatable cuff used to stop nosebleeds.

Fractional sterilization - Sterilization performed at separate intervals, usually for 15 minute periods over three to four days, so spores will develop into bacteria that can then be destroyed.

Fracture bedpan - Receptacle designed for collection of urine and feces for patients with fractures or in body casts.

Free rinsing (cleaning)- A product that will rinse away very easily or freely.

ft – Foot; feet (measure).

FTE – Full-time equivalent.

FTSG – Full thickness skin graft.

Full thickness skin graft (FTSG) – A portion of skin taken from one area of the body and placed on another area; also called skin graft.

Full-time equivalent (FTE) – The total number of employees if all employees worked full-time: total hours worked by part-time employees in one time period divided by the number of hours in a full-time position; example: if three part-time employees work a total of 48 hours in one week, and a typical full-time employee works 40 hours weekly, the FTE is 1.2 (48 hours ÷ 40 hours).

Fumigation - Disinfection by exposure to the fumes of a gaseous or vaporized disinfectant.

Functional team – A group of employees responsible for a specific function within the healthcare facility; example: CSSD personnel serve as functional team responsible for sterile processing. Within the department there are several functional teams responsible for processing components including decontamination, inspection, and assembly.

Fungicidal - A chemical that destroys fungi.

Fungicide – A substance that kills fungi.

Fungus (pl. fungi) – A type of plant-like microorganism; unicellular and multi-cellular vegetable organisms that feed on organic matter; examples: molds, mushrooms, and toadstools.

FUO – Fever of undetermined origin.

g, gm – gram.

G6PD – Glucose-6-phosphate dehydrogenase.

Gag - A device placed in the mouth to keep it open.

Gallbladder (GB) – An organ that stores and concentrates bile.

Gamma radiation - Used in radiotherapy and by some manufacturers for commercial sterilization.

Ganglion – A collection of nerve cell bodies located outside the central nervous system.

Gangrene - Death of tissue due to loss of blood supply; accompanied by bacterial invasion and putrefaction.

Gap analysis – A process that enables a healthcare facility to compare current with potential performance.

Gas – The state of matter in which molecules are practically unrestricted by cohesive forces; gas has neither shape or volume, nor is it liquid or solid.

Gas cylinder safety relief device – A device installed in a gas cylinder or container to prevent rupture of the cylinder by overpressures resulting from certain conditions of exposure; the device may be a frangible (breakable) disc, fusible plug, or relief valve.

Gasket – A pliable strip on sterilization containers that seals the lid and the container to prevent entry of microorganisms.

Gas pressure regulator – A device that may be connected to the cylinder valve outlet to regulate the gas pressure delivered to a system.

Gastrectomy - An operation to remove all or part of the stomach.

Gastric balloon - An inflatable device implanted in the stomach as an adjunct to therapy of morbid obesity.

Gastric connecting tube - Tubing used to connect a nasogastric tube to a suction collection container.

Gastric lavage tray - A collection of instruments and supplies used to irrigate or wash out the stomach to remove ingested poisons.

Gastric suction unit - A device that aspirates gastric and intestinal contents.

Gastric tube - A tube made of rubber or plastic that is inserted into the stomach.

Gastroenteritis - Inflammation of the stomach and intestines with symptoms similar to enteritis and dysentery; often caused by the enteric group of bacteria; examples: Salmonella paratyphi and Salmonella schottmuller.

Gastrointestinal (GI) - Pertaining to the stomach and intestine or the digestive tract as a whole.

Gastroscope - An endoscope designed for passage into the stomach to examine its interior.

Gastroscopy - An examination of the stomach with a gastroscope, an instrument to view the inside of the stomach.

Gauge - A standard of measurement.

Gauge pressure (steam sterilizer) - Absolute pressure (-) atmospheric pressure (14.7 pounds per square inch at sea level); also called "overpressure."

Gauze - A surgical dressing made of loosely woven cotton threads.

Gauze roller - A long strip of gauze in various sizes used to wrap around a dressing.

Gavage - Introduction of material into the stomach by means of a tube.

GB – Gallbladder.

Gene – The biological unit of heredity; self-reproducing and located in a definite position (locus) on a specific chromosome.

Generalized infection - One involving the whole body.

Genetic - Pertaining to genes or heredity.

Genitourinary (GU) – Pertaining to the genital and urinary systems.

Genus – A group of one or more related species.

Geobacillus stearothermophilus – A highly resistant but relative harmless nonpathogenic microorganism used to challenge steam and dry heat sterilizers.

Geriatrics - A branch of medicine that deals with the problems and diseases of old age and aging patients.

Germ – A microorganism that causes disease.

Germicidal - Related to destroying germs.

Germicide – An agent that kills germs.

GFR – Glomerular filtration rate.

GI – Gastrointestinal.

Gland - An organ that produces a certain substance and secretes this substance into the body.

Glaucoma – A disorder involving increased fluid pressure within the eye.

Gloves - Coverings for the hands; used to protect the patient or wearer.

Glucometer – An instrument to measure the glucose level in blood.

Glucose - Simple sugar; the main energy source for the cells; dextrose.

Glutaraldehyde - A chemical compound used in aqueous solution as a disinfectant and sterilant.

Glycerin – A liquid used as a solvent, lubricant, and sweetener.

Glycerin/lemon swab – A small wad of material used for oral hygiene.

Goal – A statement outlining the accomplishments a department or organization wishes to attain. Departmental goals are often planned to help the organization attain its goals.

Gonad - Sex gland; ovary or testis.

Gonorrhea – A contagious venereal disease of the genital mucous membranes; caused by Neisseria gonorrhoeae.

GP – General practitioner.

gr – Grain.

Graduate (measurement) - A container marked with graduations; used for liquid measurements.

Graft - Healthy skin, bone, or other tissue taken from one part of the body to replace diseased or injured tissue removed from another part of the body.

Gram – The basic unit of weight in the metric system.

Gram-negative - Losing the purple stain or decolorized by alcohol in Gram's method of staining; a primary identification characteristic of certain microorganisms.

Gram-positive - Retaining the purple stain or resisting decolorization by alcohol in Gram's method of staining.

Gram stain – A differential stain used to classify bacteria as gram-positive or gram-negative depending upon whether they retain or lose the primary stain (crystal violet) when subjected to a decolorizing agent.

Grapevine – An informal channel of communication throughout an organization.

Grasper – An instrument with jaws at working end either with teeth, serrated or atraumatic used to grasp tissue.

Gravity – The pull toward the center of the earth.

Green purchasing -- The placement of purchasing priority not only on price and quality but also on a product's impact on the environment.

Greenhouse gases – Gases in the earth's atmosphere that trap the sun's energy and keep it within the earth's atmosphere. Naturally-occurring greenhouse gases include water vapor, ozone, carbon dioxide, methane, and nitrous oxide.

Grievance – A formal employee complaint.

Grievance procedure – The process used by employees, management, and the union to resolve conflicts in a unionized facility.

Gross soil - Tissue, body fat, blood, and other body substances.

Group buying – A purchasing system in which orders for products of a specified quality are combined for participating facilities. Vendors receiving the order then deliver products to and receive payment from the participating facilities; sometimes referred to as "centralized" or "group" purchasing.

Group dynamics – The manner in which team members interact as they work together as a group and the ways that groups form, function, and dissolve.

Group interview – An interviewing method commonly used for administrative positions in which an applicant is interviewed by a small group of potential peers.

Group purchasing organization (GPO) – An organization that obtains contract pricing for high volume purchases of items with a common specification on behalf of its facility members.

GTT – Glucose tolerance test.

GU – Genitourinary.

GYN, gyn – Gynecology.

Gynecologist - A doctor specializing in gynecology.

Gynecology – The branch of medicine dealing with disease and disorders of the female reproductive system.

H

H, Hr – Hour.

HAI – Healthcare-associated infection.

Hb - Hemoglobin.

Halogen - Any of the four very active non-metallic chemical elements: chlorine, iodine, bromine, and fluorine.

Hammer - One of the three middle ear bones; attaches to the tympanic membrane.

Hand bacterial count – A method of estimating the number of bacteria present on one's hand.

Hand hygiene - The act of washing one's hands with soap and water or using an alcohol-based hand rub.

Harassment – The act of systematic and/or unwanted and annoying actions of one or more persons including threats or demands.

Harassment (sexual) – Unwanted sexual approaches and/or repeated unpleasant, degrading, and/or sexist comments made to an employee with an implied suggestion that his/her employment status, promotion, or position treatment requires a positive response (cooperation).

Hardness (water) – The amount of dissolved minerals in water that alters the effectiveness of many disinfectants, detergents, and soaps.

Harmonic scalpel - A surgical tool that uses ultrasound waves to cut tissue and seal bleeding vessels at the same time.

Hazard Communication Standard (Haz Com) – An OSHA regulation that requires chemical manufacturers, suppliers, and importers to identify and assess the hazards of their chemicals, and to communicate that information to their employees and customers with the use of Material Safety Data Sheets; see Material Safety Data Sheets.

Hazardous waste - Substances that cannot be disposed of in the facility's normal trash system.

Haz com - Hazard Communication Standard.

Hb – Hemoglobin.

HBV - Hepatitis B.

HCV – Hepatitis C.

HCFC - Hydrochlorofluorocarbon gas

Head halter - An orthopedic device used to position the head for cervical traction.

Health care - The prevention, treatment, and management of illness and the preservation of mental and physical well-being through the services offered by the medical and allied health professions.

Healthcare-associated infection (HAI) – Almost any clinically-evident infection that does not originate from the patient's original admitting diagnosis; formerly called nosocomial infection.

Healthcare facility – Any building where medical treatment is provided or medicine is practiced.

Health care products - Medical devices, medicinal products (pharmaceuticals and biologics), and in vitro diagnostics.

Health Insurance Portability and Accountability Act (HIPAA) – This act provides a rule that protects the privacy of individually identifiable health information and a patient safety rule that protects identifiable information being used to analyze patient safety events and improve patient safety.

Heart – The muscular organ that pumps blood throughout the body.

Heart-lung machine – A pump-oxygenator that temporarily assumes the functions of the heart and lungsduring open heart surgery.

Heart rate (HR) - The number ofheart beats per unit of time usually minutes.

Heat resistant - An inanimate or animate object that is generally unaffected by the application of heat.

Heat sealer – Machine designed to seal peel pouches by applying high temperatures to the open end of a paper/plastic pouch.

Heat sensitive (organism) - An organism that is readily affected or damaged by the application of heat.

Heat sink - Heat-absorbent material; a mass that readily absorbs heat.

Heat-up time - Time required for entire load to reach a pre-selected sterilizing temperature after the chamber has reached that temperature.

Heel/elbow cushion - A padded covering designed to fit over the heel or elbow for prevention of pressure sores.

Hematology - The science concerned with the study of blood, blood cells, and blood-forming tissues.

Hematoma - Swelling filled with blood.

Hematuria - Blood in the urine.

Hemiplegia - Paralysis of one side of the body; usually caused by a stroke.

Hemo - Prefix meaning blood.

Hemodialysis - Removal of impurities from the blood by passage through a semi-permeable membrane.

Hemodialyzer - Equipment used to remove impurities and waste products from blood before returning it to the patient's body.

Hemoglobin (Hb) - Iron-containing protein in red blood cells that transports oxygen.

Hemolysis - The destruction of red blood cells which leads to the release of hemoglobin from within the red blood cells into the blood plasma.

Hemolytic – The destruction of red blood cells with the liberation of hemoglobin.

Hemorrhage - Loss of blood.

Hemostasis - Stoppage of bleeding.

Hemostat - A forceps used to clamp off a blood vessel.

Hemostatic forceps – A surgical instrument used to control flow of blood.

Hepa - A filter or respirator that does not allow very fine particles to pass through it; used when caring for patients with active tuberculosis.

Heparin – A substance that prevents blood clotting; anticoagulant.

Hepatitis - Inflammation of the liver; usually caused by the hepatitis virus.

Hepatitis B (HBV) - A bloodborne pathogenic virus that can cause inflammation of the liver. An infected person can be symptomatic or asymptomatic. Symptoms include jaundice, flu-like manifestations, and liver failure. The viral incubation period can vary from 4 to 25 weeks. An effective HBV vaccine is available.

Hepatitis C (HCV) - The hepatitis C virus is transferred primarily through blood, and is more persistent than hepatitis A or B.

Heredity - Transmission of characteristics from parent to offspring by genes.

Hernia - Protrusion of an organ or tissue through the wall of the cavity in which it is normally enclosed.

Herpes simplex – A mild, acute, eruptive, vesicular virus disease of the skin and mucous membrane.

Herpes zoster - Shingles; an acute virus disease characterized by a vesicular dermatitis which follows a nerve trunk.

Hertz (Hz) – Cycles per second.

Hidden agenda – Slang term relating to a motive, objective, or plan prompting a conversation or action that is not known to others.

High efficiency particulate air filter - Special filter with minimum efficiency of 99.97%; commonly called HEPA filter.

High-level disinfection – A process that uses a sterilant for a shorter contact time than that used for sterilization and that kills all microbial organisms but not necessarily large numbers of bacterial spores.

High-vacuum steam sterilizer – A sterilizer that uses a vacuum pump to remove air from the chamber, making it faster than a gravity-displacement sterilizer to complete a sterilization cycle.

HIPAA – See Health Insurance Portability and Accountability Act.

Hippocratic oath – A document originally written by Hippocrates, an ancient scholar, that is subscribed to by physicians; addresses numerous concerns including the need to treat patients to the best of one's abilities, to preserve a patient's privacy, to teach medicine to the next generation, and to prevent disease, among others.

Histology - The study of tissues.

HIV - Human immunodeficiency virus.

HMO - Health maintenance organization.

Hold-shelf – A service offered by some instrument maintenance and repair companies that involves customized tray shipping and complete on-line billing.

Homeostasis - State of balance within the body; maintenance of body conditions within set limits.

Hormones - Chemical messengers that travel through the blood and act on target organs.

Hospice - A team-oriented approach for providing terminally-ill patient care that considers medical, physical, social, emotional, and spiritual needs of the patient; also called hospice care.

Hospital - An institution that provides medical, surgical, or psychiatric care and treatment for the sick or the injured.

Hospital alliance – A group of hospitals that shares services and information and develops group-purchasing programs to reduce costs.

Hospital quality measures (The Joint Commission) – Standardized common measures that are integral to improving the quality of care provided to hospital patients and bringing value to stakeholders by focusing on the actual results of care.

Host – An animal, plant, or human that supports the growth of microorganisms.

Hot and cold therapy device – A device that reduces swelling, pain and muscle cramps and is used to treat arthritis, pyrogenic infection, and gastrointestinal cramps. Depending on the required therapy, water is cooled or heated and then runs through a disposable pad wrapped around the area being treated. Smaller, "heat only" devices similar to electric heating pads are used on sore muscles.

Hot pack – A moist, heated dressing for therapeutic treatment.

Hourly employee (non-exempt employee) – An hourly-paid staff member who must be paid overtime under requirements of the Fair Labor Standards Act (FLSA).

HR – Heart rate.

HR – Human resources.

hr – Hour.

Huck towel – An all-cotton surgical towel with a honeycomb- effect weave.

Human immunodeficiency virus (HIV) – The virus that causes AIDS.

Human relations – The development and maintenance of effective interpersonal (between people) relationships that enhance teamwork.

Human resources (HR) – The persons employed by the healthcare facility; the department in a hospital or business that handles employment matters.

Humerus - Upper arm bone.

Humidity - The amount of water vapor in the air.

HVAC – Heating, ventilating, and air conditioning

Hx – History.

Hydration – The act of combining with water.

Hydrocarbon - Chemically identifiable compound of carbon and hydrogen.

Hydrochlorofluorocarbon gas (HCFC) – A gas that, when mixed with other gases, yields an inflammable gas.

Hydrogen ion concentration (pH) – The degree of concentration of hydrogen ions in a solution used to indicate the reaction of that solution; expressed as pH (the logarithm of the reciprocal of the hydrogen ion concentration). The pH scale is 0-14; pH of 7 is neutral (neither acid nor alkaline); pH below 7 is acid; pH above 7 is alkaline.

Hydrogen peroxide - An oxidizing and bleaching agent; also used as a sterilant for heat sensitive items in low temperature sterilizers.

Hydrologic cycle – The continual movement of water from the atmosphere to the earth and back to the atmosphere.

Hydrolysis - Splitting of large molecules by the addition of water (as in digestion).

Hydrophilic - Describing a substance that absorbs or adsorbs water.

Hydrophobic - Describing a substance that does not absorb or adsorb water.

Hygiene - A science of the establishment and maintenance of health.

Hyperglycemia – An abnormal increase in the amount of glucose in the blood.

Hypertension - High blood pressure.

Hyperthermia - High fever; producing heat by physical means.

Hyperthermia unit - A device designed to pump heated or cooled water through a coiled pad to therapeutically raise or lower body temperature.

Hypertonic – A solution with a higher osmotic pressure than that of a reference solution.

Hypodermic needle - A hollow needle used for injections or for obtaining fluid specimens.

Hypoglycemia – An abnormal decrease in the amount of glucose in the blood.

Hypotension - Low blood pressure.

Hypothermia - Abnormally low body temperature.

Hypothermia unit – A device that pumps heated or cooled water through a coiled pad to therapeutically raise or lower body temperature.

Hypotonic – A solution which is of less than isotonic concentration.

Hypoxia - Reduced oxygen supply to the tissues.

Hysterectomy - An operation in which the uterus and cervix are removed.

Hz – Hertz; a unit of measurement relating to cycles per second.

I & D –Irrigation & debridement.

I & O – Intake and output.

IM – Intramuscular.

IABP – Intra-aortic balloon pump.

IAHCSMM - International Association of Healthcare Central Service Materiel Management.

IBP – Intravenous blood pressure.

Ice pack - A rubber or plastic bag filled with ice to produce cold.

ICF – Intracellular fluid.

ICS – Intercostal space.

Icteric - Yellow pigmentation of the tissues, membranes, and secretions caused by the deposit of bile pigment; usually a sign of liver or gall bladder disease.

ICU – Intensive Care Unit.

ICRA - Infection control risk assessment.

Idiopathic - Of unknown cause.

Idiosyncrasy - Individual and peculiar susceptibility or sensitivity to a drug, protein, or other matter.

IDN - Integrated delivery network.

IM – Intermedullary.

Implants - Artificial substitutes for body parts, and materials inserted into tissue for functional, cosmetic, or therapeutic purposes. Implants, all surgically inserted or grafted into the body, tend to be used therapeutically.

Ileostomy - An opening created by a surgeon into the ileum, part of the small intestine, from the outside of the body. An ileostomy provides a new path for waste material to leave the body after part of the intestine has been removed.

Ileostomy appliance – A device used to fit over a stoma for fecal collection.

Ileum – The last portion of the small intestine.

Image intensifier – Medical equipment that uses low-intensity X-rays to produce an image shown on a video screen.

Immune - Exempt from a given infection.

Immunity – The power of an individual to resist or overcome the effects of a particular disease or other harmful agent.

Immunization – The process of conferring immunity on an individual.

Impact marker – A tool which engraves with a forceful impact that indents and "breaks" the polished metal surface leaving an inscribed marking.

Impervious - Material that resists fluids, especially body fluids, such as gowns, aprons, and surgical drapes.

Impingement – The spray-force action of pressurized water against instruments being processed to physically remove bioburden.

Implode - Bursting inward.

Implosion - Bursting inward; the opposite of an explosion; occurs when cavitations in an energized solution collapse.

In vitro - Referring to a process or reaction carried out in a culture test tube or Petri dish.

In vivo - In the living body.

Inactivation - To stop or destroy activity.

Inanimate - Not endowed with life or spirit; not alive.

Incipient - Just beginning.

Incision - A cut made by a knife, especially for surgical purposes.

Incompatible - Not capable of being mixed without undergoing destructive chemical changes or antagonism.

Incontinent pad - Material placed under a patient to collect any drainage or excrement.

Incubate - To maintain under optimum environmental conditions favorable for growth.

Incubation period – The period between when infection occurs and appearance of the first symptoms.

Incubator (infant) - A medical device consisting of an enclosed, heated plexi-glass bed in which environmental conditions including light, temperature and humidity are fully controlled; used for premature infants.

Incubator (microorganisms) - Apparatus for maintaining a constant and suitable temperature for the growth and cultivation of microorganisms.

Indefinite shelf life – The shelf life of hospital-sterilized items without a definite expiration date; based on premise that shelf life is event- not time-related. The user must assure the integrity of the packaging is intact, clean, and properly identified.

Indemnification – The act of reimbursing for a loss.

Indicator (quality) – A measurable variable which relates to the outcome of patient care or employee safety.

Indicator - See specific indicator: biological, chemical, mechanical.

Indirect contact – The transfer of infection by means including inanimate objects, contaminated fingers, water, and food.

Induction – The process by which new CSSD employees are oriented to departmental policies and procedures.

In-dwelling (catheter) - Held in place within a part of the body, especially in the bladder.

inf. – Inferior.

Infant incubator – A device that creates and controls the environment of newborns; see incubator (infant).

Infant warmer - A medical apparatus that consists of an open bed with an overhead warmer and used to keep an infant warm; also called radiant warmer.

Infarct – An area of tissue damaged from lack of blood supply caused by blockage of a vessel.

Infection - Invasion of body tissue by microorganisms which multiply and produce a reaction.

Infection control - Control of active infectious disease; requires (a) working knowledge of the usefulness and applications of physical and chemical agents that suppress or kill microorganisms and (b) familiarity with the sources of potentially dangerous microorganisms, routes by which they spread, and their portals of entry into the body.

Infection control risk assessment (ICRA) process – A multi-disciplinary process that focuses on reducing risk from infection throughout planning, design, and construction (including renovation) activities undertaken by a healthcare facility.

Infection prevention – Procedures that reduce the incidence of infections.

Infectious - Having the ability to transmit disease.

Infectious waste - Waste that potentially contains sufficient numbers of pathogens with sufficient virulence so that exposure into a susceptible host could result in an infectious disease.

Inferior - Below or lower.

Infestation - Lodgment, development, and reproduction of arthropods on a body or clothing.

Inflammation - Reaction of the tissues to an injury; a protective mechanism to an irritant on tissues.

Informed consent (patient) – The process by which a person learns key information about a medical event including benefits and risks before deciding whether to participate in a treatment, non-treatment, or procedure.

Infrastructure (information system) – Components including hardware, software, databases, telecommunications networks, and procedures that comprise an information system.

Infusion - The continuous slow introduction of a solution into a vein.

Infusion pump - A device used to infuse fluids, medication or nutrients into a patient's circulatory system in a controlled manner; generally used intravenously, although subcutaneous, arterial, and epidural infusions are occasionally used.

Infusion therapy – Relates to the introduction of fluid other than blood into a vein; also called intravenous (IV) therapy.

ING – Inguinal.

Inguinal (ING) - Of, pertaining to, or situated in the groin.

Inhibition - Checking or restraining.

Injection - To introduce a substance into the body.

Inoculate - To implant or introduce causative agents of disease into an animal or plant or microbes onto culture media.

Inoculated carrier - Carrier on which a defined number of test organisms has been deposited.

Inoculation - The intentional introduction of certain organisms into the body to protect against subsequent infection.

Inorganic - Composed of matter other than plant or animal: minerals.

Inpatient care unit – A unit that provides care for patients admitted to a facility for treatment requiring at least one overnight stay.

Insecticide - An agent that destroys insects.

In-service training – Training program designed to enhance existing skills or to teach new skills that may be delivered in off-or on-job locations.

Inspect - To view closely in critical appraisal.

Installation qualification (IQ) - Obtaining and documenting evidence that equipment has been provided and installed in accordance with its specifications.

Instrument - Utensil or implement.

Instrument tracking system - A computer-assisted program for tracking instruments, report generation and staff productivity monitoring.

Instrument washer sterilizer (IWS) - Combination units that wash and sterilize instruments to insure the safety of processing personnel.

Insubordination – The willful disobedience of a request or directive from a higher-level manager.

Insufflator - A device used to treat medically by blowing a powder, gas, or vapor into a bodily cavity.

Insulin – A hormone that reduces the level of sugar in the blood.

Integrated delivery network (IDN) – A system of healthcare providers and organizations which provide (or arrange to provide) a coordinated range of services to a specific population.

Integrating indicator – A chemical indicator designed to react to all critical parameters over a specified range of sterilization cycles and whose performance has been correlated to the performance of the relevant biological indicator (BI) under the labeled conditions of use.

Intensive care unit (ICU) - A specialized section of a hospital that provides comprehensive and continuous care for persons who are critically ill and who can benefit from treatment.

Intercellular - Between cells.

Intercostal space (ICS) – The space between two adjacent ribs.

Interface – The connection between two computer systems through which information is exchanged.

Interface engine application – A computer program that stores, forwards, maps, and routes data between various systems within a healthcare facility.

Intermediate-level disinfection – The process that utilizes an agent to kill viruses, mycobacteria, fungi, and vegetative bacteria but not bacterial spores.

Intermittent (fractional) sterilization - Destruction of microorganisms by moist heat for given periods of time on several successive days to allow spores during the rest periods to germinate into vegetative forms (which are most easily destroyed).

Intermittent positive-pressure breathing - The active inflation of the lungs during inhalation under positive pressure from a cycling valve.

Intermittent suction device - A suction device that starts and stops suctioning at periodic intervals.

Internal - On the inside.

Internal audit – The process of conducting a within-organization examination of one or more departments or organizational processes.

Internal construction – Renovation and/or new construction that involves the interior of the Central Service department or the healthcare facility.

International System of Units (SI) – The modern form of the metric system.

International unit (IU) - A unit of biological material such as enzymes, hormones, and vitamins established by the International Conference for the Unification of Formulas.

Internet – A cooperative message-forwarding system that links computer networks throughout the world.

Interstitial - Between; pertaining to spaces or structures in an organ between active tissues.

Interview – A face-to-face meeting with an individual in which questions are asked and responded to; examples include applicant interviews to assess employment suitability and appraisal interviews to evaluate job performance.

Intra-aortic balloon pump - A medical device that uses a balloon catheter to augment the functioning of a severely weakened heart. The catheter is placed in the aorta and is inflated and deflated in synchronization with the patient's heartbeat.

Intracatheter - A plastic tube inserted within a vein for infusion, injection, or monitoring.

Intracellular - Within a cell or cells.

Intracellular fluid (ICF) – Fluid that is within cells.

Intranet – A network consisting only of computers for a single organization that can be at the same or different locations.

Intraoperative radiation therapy (IORT) –A protocol that delivers a concentrated beam of radiation to cancerous tumors while they are exposed during surgery.

Intrapreneur – A creative and innovative person within a large organization who is directly responsible for successfully managing an aspect of the organization's business.

Intrauterine device (IUD) - A small object inserted through the cervix and placed in the uterus to prevent pregnancy.

Intravenous (IV) - Within or into the veins.

Intravenous blood pressure (IBP) - A method of measuring blood pressure internally by using a sensitive IV catheter inserted into an artery to provide a more accurate reading.

Intravenous pyelogram (IVP) - An x-ray examination of the kidneys, ureters, and urinary bladder that uses iodinated contrast material injected into veins.

Intravenous urography (IVU) - An x-ray procedure used to assess problems in the kidneys, ureters, bladder, and urethra.

Intubate - The introduction of a tube into a hollow organ.

Intubation - The process of inserting a breathing tube into the throat down to the trachea. This tube is connected to an ambu bag, respirator, or ventilator which pushes measured amounts of air into the lungs and lets it out again to assist the patient with breathing.

In-use testing - Evaluation of infection-control chemicals, aseptic techniques, and sanitary and sterilization procedures under actual working conditions.

Invalid ring - An inflatable plastic or rubber ring used to relieve sacral pressure.

Inventory - Reusable equipment and consumable items used to provide healthcare services for patients.

Inventory (consumable) - Assets such as wrapping supplies, processing chemicals, and other items which are consumed as healthcare services are provided to patients.

Inventory (control) – Procedures to maintain appropriate quantities of supplies to support patient care activities.

Inventory (official) - Consumable products found in Central Service and other storerooms, warehouses, and satellite storage areas; included as an asset on a healthcare facility's balance sheet.

Inventory (physical) – Products stored in a healthcare facility's supply system; also the procedure used to determine the quantity and cost of inventory on hand at a specific point in time.

Inventory (reusable) - Relatively inexpensive assets such as medical devices and sterilization containers that can be reused as healthcare services are provided to patients.

Inventory service level – The percentage of items filled (available) when an order is placed.

Inventory stock out rate – The percentage of items that cannot be filled (are not available) when an order is placed.

Inventory turnover rate - Number of times per year (or other time period) that inventory is purchased, consumed, and replaced.

Inventory (unofficial) - Consumable products found in user areas such as surgical locations and labs. Unofficial inventory has usually been expensed to user units and is stored in various locations on the units.

Invoice – A payment request by a vendor for products sold or services provided.

Invoice (payment method) – A method of paying vendor bills on a by-delivery basis; the amount specified by the delivery invoice is paid at or before the time specified in the invoice.

Iodoform - A yellow crystalline, volatile compound with a penetrating, persistent odor used in an antiseptic dressing.

Iodophor – A disinfectant that is a combination of iodine and a solubilizing agent (or a carrier) which slowly liberates or releases free iodine when diluted with water.

Ion – An electronically-charged particle formed by the loss or gain of one or more electrons.

Ionize - To dissociate into ions or to become electrically charged.

IORT – Intraoperative radiation therapy.

IQ - Installation qualification.

Iris – The circular colored region of the eye around the pupil.

Irrigation - The washing of a body cavity or surface by flowing solution which is inserted and then removed.

Ischemia - Lack of blood supply to an area.

Islets - Groups of cells in the pancreas that produce hormones; Islets of Langerhans.

ISO 9000 - International standards used by participating organizations to help assure that they consistently deliver quality services and products.

Isolate - To place by itself; to separate from others.

Isolation - To set apart or quarantine a patient with a communicable disease from others.

Isolette - An incubator.

Isotonic – A solution having the same osmotic pressure as that of another solution taken as a standard reference.

Isotope – A form of an element with the same atomic number as another but with a different atomic weight.

Issue (product) – The task of transferring items from storage areas to user departments in quantities that enable user personnel to meet production needs.

Issue requisition – A document used to identify the products and their quantities removed from storage areas when formal inventory control procedures are used.

IU – International unit.

IUD – Intrauterine device.

IV – Intravenous.

IVP – Intravenous pyelogram.

IVU – Intravenous urography.

J

Jargon - Specialized words or phrases known only by persons working in a position.

Jaundice - Excess of bile pigments in blood, skin, and mucous membranes with a resulting yellow appearance of the individual.

Jaw - Either of two or more opposable parts that open and close for holding or crushing something between them.

TJC – The Joint Commission.

Jejunum – The second portion of the small intestine.

Jelly lubricant - A water-soluble lubricant used to facilitate the introduction of catheters and tubes.

JIT - Just in time.

Job analysis – The process of gathering, examining, and interpreting information about specific job tasks for a new position or for tasks in an existing position that have changed.

Job classification – A group of positions with similar duties and responsibilities that justifies a common name and similar treatment for selection, compensation, and other human resource purposes.

Job code – Identification numbers assigned to specific jobs within a facility.

Job description - A human resources tool that identifies the major tasks performed by persons in specific positions.

Job evaluation – A process that compares jobs to determine appropriate pay rates.

Job offer – A written proposal by an employer to a prospective employee that specifies employment terms; a legally valid acceptance of the offer creates a binding employee contract.

Job satisfaction – A measurement that assesses how employees feel about their work environment, pay, benefits, and other job-related factors.

Job shadowing – An unpaid work experience in which new employees or students learn about a job by following an experienced employee during a work shift.

Job sharing – The situation in which two employees share hours and perform the work required for one full-time position.

Job specification – A list of personal requirements judged necessary for someone to successfully work in a position.

Joint - Any place where two bones meet.

Joint Commission - A regulatory organization whose purpose is to encourage the attainment of uniformly high standards of institutional medical care, establish guidelines for the operation of hospitals and other health care facilities, and conduct survey and accreditation programs (See The Joint Commission).

JRA – Juvenile rheumatoid arthritis.

Julian calendar - A calendar introduced in Rome in 46 B.C. establishing the 12-month year of 365 days, with each fourth year (called a "leap" year) having 366 days, and the months each having 31 or 30 days, except for February with only 28 days or, in leap years, 29 days.

Julian date - The Julian day or Julian day number is the number of days that have elapsed since January 1 of a specific year.

Jury trial – A trial of a lawsuit in which the case is presented to a jury, and the factual questions and judgment are determined by the jury.

Just cause – The underlying principle that an employer must have reasonable justification for disciplining an employee and that the discipline is not arbitrary, capricious (impulsive), or discriminatory.

Just in time (JIT) - A method of inventory distribution where a vendor holds inventory for an organization and delivers items on a regular basis which go directly to supply carts.

K

K – Potassium.

Kelly hemostatic forceps - An instrument used for grasping.

Key performance indicator (KPI) – A measurable assessment factor such as item accuracy, case carts per technician, and sterilization accuracy.

kg – kilogram.

Kick bucket - A medical receptacle, usually stainless steel and mounted on wheels and easily moved around the operating room by the foot. Disposable articles used to absorb blood or fluids during the procedure are tossed into the buckets placed about the operating room. At the end of the procedure, the sponges in the bucket are countered to ensure that all counts are correct.

Kidneys - Organs that remove excess water and waste substances from the blood in a process that yields urine.

Killing power – The ability of a chemical to kill bacteria under laboratory conditions and during in-use testing.

Knee supporter - An elastic binder used to support a weak or injured knee.

KO – Keep open.

KUB – Kidneys, ureters, and bladder; an X-ray of the kidney, ureter, and bladder.

L

l – Liter.

L/LT – Left.

Labeling – A legend, work, or mark attached to, included in, belonging to, or accompanying any medical device.

Labor intensive – The need for people rather than equipment or technology to perform required work tasks.

Labor-management contract – A binding agreement between a labor union and management that governs covered employees' wages, benefits, and other working conditions.

Laceration - A torn and ragged wound.

Lacrimal - Referring to tears or the tear glands.

Lactated ringer's solution – A mixture used for fluid and electrolyte replacement.

Lactation - Secretion of milk.

Lactic acid – An organic acid that accumulates in muscle cells functioning without oxygen.

LAD – Left anterior descending coronary artery

Laissez-faire (leadership style) – A leadership approach that minimizes directing employees and, instead, maximizes the delegation of tasks to staff members.

LAM – Laminectomy

Lamina - Two broad plates that fuse to complete the roof of the vertebral arch.

Laminar airflow - Filtered air moving along separate parallel flow planes to surgical suites, nurseries, bacteriology work areas, and pharmacies; prevents collection of bacterial contamination or hazardous chemical fumes in work areas.

Laminectomy (LAM)– A spinal operation to remove the lamina, a part of the vertebral bone.

LAN – Local area network.

Lancet - A sterile, sharp, pointed blade which can be used to perform a capillary puncture.

Lap – Laparoscopy.

Lap sponge - Gauze used during surgical procedures to control bleeding and protect tissues; contains a radiopaque element for detection.

Laparoflator - A type of medical insufflator which is inserted through a small incision in the abdomen during an investigative surgical procedure and used to maintain constant intra-abdominal pressure in the patient.

Laparoscope - A long, slender optical instrument for insertion through the abdominal wall used to visualize the interior of the peritoneal cavity.

Laparoscopic assisted vaginal hysterectomy (LAVH) - A procedure used to remove the uterus, Fallopian tubes, and/or ovaries through the vagina.

Laparoscopy (Lap) - A minimally invasive surgical technique in which a lighted scope (laparoscope) is inserted into a small incision in the abdomen; commonly used to visualize the inside of the abdomen for diagnosis, to retrieve tissue samples for biopsy, and to perform surgical procedures using tiny instruments passed into the abdomen through tiny incisions.

Laparotomy – A surgical procedure that allows the doctor to inspect the organs in the abdomen

Large intestine – The digestive organ that dehydrates digestive residues (feces); also called colon.

Laryngoscope - A small, hand-held medical device that consists of a handle, a tongue depressor, and a light source; normally used to move aside the patient's tongue and open the throat and expose the larynx so the doctor can insert a breathing tube or perform other procedures.

Laryngectomy - A surgical procedure to remove all or part of the larynx.

Laryngoscopy - Examination of the larynx with a mirror (indirect laryngoscopy) or with a laryngoscope (direct laryngoscopy).

Larynx - Voice box.

Laser – A device that produces a very intense beam of light used in some types of surgery to cut or destroy tissue.

lat – lateral.

Latching mechanism – A mechanical device that secures a rigid sterilization container's lid to the container's bottom.

Latent heat - Additional heat required to change the state of a substance from solid to liquid at its melting point, or from liquid to gas at its boiling point, after the temperature of the substance has reached either of these points.

Lateral - Farther from the midline; toward the side.

Lateral violence – A situation that occurs when people are victims of dominance and then confront each other rather than the system that oppresses them.

Latex – A common form of rubber used in the manufacture of hospital and medical supplies.

Latex sensitivity - Sensitivity (allergic reaction) of some persons to latex caused by exposure to latex that is improperly processed; symptoms range from skin rash, primarily on the hands, to anaphylactic reaction.

LAVH – Laparoscopic assisted vaginal hysterectomy

Lawsuit – A common term for a legal action by one person or entity against another person or entity.

Layoff – The termination of employees and/or the elimination of jobs during organizational restructuring.

lb – Pound

Leader – A person who influences and guides others towards the achievement of goals.

Leadership – The process by which an individual identifies a goal, outlines a process, influences a group, and directs its members towards attainment of the goal.

Leadership development – Formal or informal training programs designed for management-level employees that facilitate the development of leadership skills and styles required for their position.

Leak test (endoscope) – An endoscope processing procedure that ensures the device's flexible covering and internal channels are watertight.

Learning styles – The way a person likes to learn; examples: visual, auditory, and tactile.

Leg bag - A plastic urinary drainage bag connected to a urinary catheter.

Lens – The biconvex structure of the eye that changes in thickness to accommodate near and far vision; crystalline lens.

Lens paper - A special nonabrasive material used to clean optical lenses.

Lesion – A wound or local injury; a specific change or morphological alteration by disease or injury.

Lethal - Pertaining to death.

Leukemia – A malignant blood disease characterized by abnormal development of white blood cells.

Leukocyte - White blood cell.

Levin tube – A hollow tube used for gastric and intestinal aspiration or tube feeding.

LG –Large.

LH – Luteinizing hormone.

Liability (accounting) – The value of obligations owed by the organization.

Ligament - A band of connective tissue that connects a bone to another bone.

Limb holder - A canvas device used to support an arm or leg.

Line balancing and capacity analysis/assessment – A tool that helps to analyze process work flow by determining the ability of the CSSD to meet customers' needs.

Line managers – Department heads, managers, supervisors, and other decision-makers in the healthcare facility's chain of command.

Line-level employees – Staff members whose jobs are considered entry-level or non-supervisory and who are paid an hourly rate rather than a salary.

Linen pack - Linens packaged together to be used for draping or donning by staff, usually for surgical procedures.

Lipid virus - A virus whose core is surrounded by a coat of lipoprotein; generally easily inactivated by many types of disinfectants including low-level disinfectants.

Lipids - Group of fats or fatty substances characterized by insolubility in water.

Lipoprotein – A protein-coated package that carries fat and cholesterol through the bloodstream.

Liposuction - A cosmetic surgery procedure that removes fat from many different areas of the human body including the abdomen, neck, thighs, buttocks, arms, and more.

Liquid-proof - Material that prevents the penetration of liquids and microorganisms.

Liquid-resistant - Material that inhibits the penetration of liquids.

Liter - Basic unit of volume in metric system.

Lithotripsy - A minimally invasive procedure that uses sound waves to break up a kidney or other stone into smaller pieces so they can pass out of the urinary system.

Litigation – A legal proceeding in a court of law.

Litigious society – A society in which people tend to engage in lawsuits, see lawsuit.

Liver – The organ that filters the blood to remove amino acids and neutralize some harmful toxins.

LLQ – Left lower quadrant.

Load configuration - All attributes defining the presentation of products to the sterilization process including (a) orientation of products within the primary package (b) quantity and orientation of primary packages(s) within secondary and tertiary packages (c) quantity, orientation, and placement of tertiary packages on sterilizer pallets or within carriers and (d) quantity and placement of the pallets (or carriers) within the vessel or area.

Load control number - Label information on sterilization packages, trays, or containers that identifies the sterilizer, cycle run, and date of sterilization.

Loaner instrumentation -- An instrument or set borrowed from a vendor for a scheduled or emergency surgical procedure that will be returned to the vendor following its use.

Local area network (LAN) – A network that connects several near-by computers so they can share files and devices such as printers; see network.

Local exhaust hood – A system that captures contaminated air and conducts it into an exhaust duct; also called venting hood.

Local infection – An infection confined to a restricted area.

Logarithm – An exponent indicating the power to which a fixed number (the base) must be raised to produce a given number.

Logistics – Activities designed to best assure that the correct quantity of the correct products are at the correct place at the correct time, and that they were moved there at the lowest possible cost.

Logistics (within facility) – Processes used to plan for and control products, equipment, supplies, and other items as they are purchased, stored, processed, placed into finished inventory, and/or transported throughout a healthcare facility.

Logistics management – The practice of planning and implementing the cost-effective flow of raw products, in-process inventory, and finished products from product source to product user while satisfying customer requirements.

Long-range budget – A budget that estimates expenses and revenue, if applicable, over a three, five, or even ten year time frame.

Lot (load) control number – Numbers and/or letters by which a specific group of products can be traced to a particular manufacturing or sterilization operation.

Low-level disinfection – A process that utilizes an agent to kill vegetative forms of bacteria, some fungi, and lipid viruses.

LUM/LAM – lumbar laminectomy.

Lumbar laminectomy (LUM/LAM) – A surgical procedure most often performed to treat leg pain related to herniated discs, spinal stenosis, and related conditions.

Lumbar vertebrae - The largest segments of the movable part of the vertebral column.

Lumen – The interior path through a needle, tube, or surgical instrument.

Lungs – The organs of respiration.

Lumpectomy - Surgery to remove only the cancerous breast lump.

LUQ – left upper quadrant.

Lux - One-tenth of a foot candle.

LV –Left ventricle.

Lymph - Fluid in the lymphatic system.

Lymphangiogram - An injection of a contrast medium into the lymphatic channels to take an x-ray photograph.

Lymphatic system - Series of tiny vessels throughout the body that carry lymph fluid to protect the body against disease.

Lymphocyte - White blood cell involved in antibody production.

M

M – Male.

m – Meter, minim.

M – Molar.

Macromolecules - Large molecules (proteins, carbohydrates, lipids, and nucleic acids) within a microorganism.

Macroscopic - Visible to the naked eye.

Magnet status - Award given by the American Nurses Credentialing Center to hospitals that satisfy factors measuring the strength and quality of nursing care.

Magnetic resonance imaging (MRI) - Method for studying tissue based on nuclear movement following exposure to radio waves in a powerful magnetic field.

Mainframe (computer) – A high performance computer used for large-volume computing purposes that services numerous (even hundreds) of computers at the same time; also called enterprise server.

Maintenance - A program for controlling and keeping equipment in good working condition.

Maintenance insurance – An equipment outsourcing alternative in which a hospital retains control of its equipment but contracts with an insurance organization to manage and insure the costs involved in maintaining it.

Make (do) or buy analysis – A systematic process to determine whether products should be manufactured on-site or purchased from an external supply source. Sometimes called "Do/Buy Analysis" when on-site versus vendor-provided services are analyzed.

Malaise - Indisposition, discomfort, or feeling of ill health.

Malecot catheter – A device with a particular retaining mechanism used for drainage of the body cavities, especially for suprapubic urinary drainage.

Malignant - Describing a tumor that spreads or a disorder that becomes worse and causes death.

Malleability (instrument) – The ability of a material to be worked, hammered, or shaped without breaking.

Malnutrition - State resulting from lack of food, lack of an essential component of the diet, or faulty use of food in the diet.

Malpractice - A dereliction from professional duty or a failure to exercise an accepted degree of professional skill.

Mammectomy – See mastectomy.

Mammogram – An X-ray photograph of the breast, sometimes with contrast medium injected into the breast.

Mammoplasty - Plastic repair of the breast to enlarge, reduce, or reconstruct after surgical removal of a tumor.

Managed care – Numerous techniques implemented to reduce the cost of providing healthcare and to improve its quality.

Management – The process of using what one has (resources) to accomplish goals and objectives.

Manager – One who directs the work of supervisors.

Mandible - Lower jaw bone.

Manip – Manipulation.

Mantoux test - Tuberculin skin test.

Manufacturer – A company that transforms raw materials into finished products; example, raw metals into surgical instruments.

Martensitic (stainless steel) - Metal also known as 400 series stainless steel that is magnetic and may be heat-hardened.

Mask - A protective covering worn on the face over the nose and mouth.

Mastectomy - Removal of the breast; mammectomy.

Master budget – An itemized forecast or predication of the healthcare facility's revenue and expenses for a specific time period.

Mastication - Act of chewing.

Material Safety Data Sheet (MSDS) – A written statement provided by the manufacturer of the chemical or toxic substance to the buyer of the product that provides detailed information about a chemical or toxic substance including the potential hazards of and best ways to handle a chemical or toxic substance. MSDS sheets also include information on how to treat an exposure to the chemical or toxic substance.

Materiel Management Department - Healthcare department responsible for researching, ordering, receiving, and managing inventory (consumable supplies).

Mayo stand - A portable stand or table used to provide easy access to surgical instruments and supplies during a procedure.

MCH – Mean corpuscular hemoglobin.

MCHC – Mean corpuscular hemoglobin concentration.

MCV – Mean corpuscular volume.

MD – Medical doctor.

MD - Muscular dystrophy.

Measles - Rubella; an acute, infectious virus disease characterized by fever, catarrh, coryza, Koplik spots on buccal mucous membrane, and a papular rash.

MEC - Minimum effective concentration.

Mechanical indicators - Devices built into a machine used in identifying and preventing malfunctions and operational errors.

Medial - Nearer the midline of the body.

Mediastinoscopy - A procedure in which the doctor inserts a tube into the chest to view the organs in the mediastinum. The tube is inserted through an incision above the breastbone.

Mediastinum - Region between the lungs and the organs and the vessels it contains.

Mediation – A negotiation and decision-making process in which a disinterested third party assists individuals in finding a non-binding resolution to an issue.

Medicaid - Federal and state assistance program paying covered medical expenses for low-income persons.

Medical air - Clean compressed air that can be used for patient ventilation.

Medical analyses (profession) - The health profession concerned with the performance of laboratory technology used in the diagnosis and treatment of disease as well as in health maintenance.

Medical device - Any instrument, apparatus, appliance, material or other article, used alone or in combination, including software necessary for its proper application intended by the manufacturer to be used for human beings for (a) diagnosis, prevention, monitoring, treatment, or alleviation of disease (b) diagnosis, monitoring, treatment, alleviation of, or compensation for an injury or handicap (c) investigation, replacement, or modification of the anatomy or of a physiological process or (d) control of conception.

Medical gas - Any gaseous substance that meets medical purity standards and has application in a medical environment such as oxygen, nitrous oxide and air.

Medicare – A federal medical insurance program that primarily serves those over 65 years of age regardless of income, and younger disabled persons and dialysis patients. Medical bills are paid from trust funds into which covered persons have paid.

MedWatch Program - Safety information and adverse event reporting system that serves healthcare professionals and the public by reporting serious problems suspected to be associated with the drugs and medical devices they prescribe, dispense, or use.

Membrane - Thin sheet of tissue.

Memory – The inherent ability of a substance to return to its original shape and contours.

Meningitis - Inflammation of the meninges.

Menopause – The time at which menstruation ceases.

Menses - Monthly flow of blood from the female reproductive tract.

Menstruation - Discharge of blood and tissue from the uterus normally occurring every 28 days.

Mentor – A senior employee of the healthcare facility who provides advice and counsel to less experienced staff members about matters relating to the job, facility, and profession.

Mentoring – A formal or informal relationship in which an experienced staff member provides advice and counsel to a less-experienced staff member.

mEq – Milliequivalent

Merit pay (pay for performance) – A compensation system in which pay increases are determined by an employee's performance.

Mesentery – The membranous peritoneal ligament that attaches the small intestine to the dorsal abdominal wall.

Mesophiles - Bacteria that grow best at moderate temperatures: 68°F-113°F (20°C-45°C).

Metabolic rate – The rate at which energy is released from nutrients in the cells.

Metabolism - Total chemical changes by which the nutritional and functional activities of an organism are maintained.

Metacarpals - Hand bones.

Metallurgy - Science and technology of metals.

Metastasis - Spread of tumor cells.

Metatarsals - Bones of the foot.

Meter - Basic unit of length in the metric system.

Methicillin resistant staphylococcus aureus (MRSA) – Staphylococcus aureus bacteria that have developed a resistance to Methicillin, the treatment drug of choice; usually occurs with patients who have had antibiotic therapy for a long time.

Mg – Magnesium.

mg – Milligram.

Microaerophils - Microorganisms that require free oxygen for their growth but in an amount less than that of the oxygen in the atmosphere.

Microbes - Organisms of microscopic or sub-microscopic size generally including viruses, rickettsiae, bacteria, algae, yeasts, and molds.

Microbiology – The study of microorganisms; the science which treats the nature, life, and action of microorganisms.

Microdrip - An intravenous adaptor with a drop control that emits a drop 1/10 the size of a regular drop.

Micron - Unit of measurement; 1/1000 of a millimeter or 1/25,000 of an inch or one millionth of a meter; note: one meter equals 39.37 inches.

Microorganisms - Forms of life that are too small to see with the naked eye. Bacteria, viruses, and fungi are types of microorganisms; also called "germs" and "microbes."

Microscope – An optical instrument consisting of a lens or combination of lenses for making enlarged images of minute objects.

Micturition - Passing of urine; urination.

Midbrain - Upper portion of the brain stem.

Midstream urine - A urine sample collected in the middle of voiding.

Mil - Unit of length or thickness equal to .001 of an inch.

Millosmole - One thousandth (10-3) of an osmole.

Min/max - Minimum/maximum (purchasing system)

Mineral – An inorganic substance; diet element needed in small amounts for health.

Minimally invasive surgery - A surgical procedure that uses small surgical incisions or no cuts at all and greatly reduces the amount of bleeding; examples include lithotripsy in which sound waves are used to break up a kidney or other stone without any incision required, and endoscopy which uses small scopes inserted into small cuts or body openings.

Minimum effective concentration (MEC) - Percentage concentration of the active ingredient in a disinfectant or chemical sterilant that is the minimum concentration at which the chemical meets all label claims for activity against specific microorganisms.

Minimum-maximum (purchasing system) – A system to calculate product purchase quantities that considers the minimum quantity below which inventory levels should not fall and the maximum quantity above which inventory levels should not rise.

Minimum recommended concentration (MRC) – The minimum concentration at which the manufacturer tested the product and validated its performance.

Mission – A planning tool that broadly identifies what a healthcare facility or a department within it wants to accomplish and how it plans to do so.

Mitosis - Cell division that produces two daughter cells exactly like the parent cell.

Mitral valve - Valve between the left atrium and left ventricle of the heart; bicuspid valve.

Mixed culture - Growth of two or more microorganisms in the same medium.

Mixed infection - Simultaneous process of two or more microorganisms causing an infection.

Mixture - Blend of two or more substances.

ml – Milliliter.

MI – Myocardial infarction.

mm – Millimeter.

mo – Month.

Mode of transmission (chain of infection) - Method of transfer of an infectious agent from the reservoir to a susceptible host.

Moisture sensitive - Unable to withstand dampness.

Molds - See fungus.

Molecular attraction - Adhesive forces exerted between the surface molecules of two bodies in contact.

Molecule - Smallest quantity of matter that can exist in a free state and retain all of its properties.

Monel - A trademark used for an alloy of nickel, copper, iron, and manganese.

Monitor - To systematically check or test to control the concentration of a specific ingredient or the execution of a process; may include qualitative and/or quantitative measurements.

Monopolar electrocautery - One of the two types of electrocautery. Electrical current is passed from the probe (active electrode) where cauterization occurs, and the patient's body serves as a ground. A grounding pad (returning electrode) is placed on the person's body, usually the thigh to return the current to the machine.

Monorail system – A movable vehicle that travels over rails and is used to transport products and materials between locations; example: a dumb waiter (small elevator) that moves items vertically.

Montgomery straps - Adhesive strips used to hold dressing in place; the dressing can be changed without removing the strips.

Morale – The total of one's feelings about his or her employer, work environment, peers, and other aspects of the employment.

Morgue - An area where bodies of deceased persons are kept until identified and claimed by relatives or released for burial.

Motion (legal) – A formal request made to a judge for an order or a judgment.

Motivation (extrinsic) – An inner drive motivated by external factors that may be beyond one's control.

Motivation (intrinsic) – An inner drive toward an emotionally pleasurable experience in which one accepts responsibility for the outcomes.

Mouth - The opening through which air, food, and beverages enter the body; beginning of the alimentary canal.

MRC - Minimum recommended concentration.

MRI - Magnetic resonance imaging.

MRSA - Methicillin resistant staphylococcus aureus.

MS – Multiple sclerosis.

MS - Morphine sulfate.

MSDS – Material safety data sheet.

MSH – Melanocyte-stimulating hormone.

Mucosa - Lining membrane that produces mucus; mucous membrane.

Mucous – A thick protective fluid secreted by mucous membranes and glands.

Mucous membrane - Membrane lining all body cavities that open externally including mouth.

Multiparameter indicator – An indicator designed for two or more critical parameters that indicates exposure to a sterilization cycle at stated values of the parameters.

Murmur - Abnormal heart sound.

Muslin – A broad term describing a wide variety of plain-weave cotton or cotton/polyester fabrics with approximately 140 threads per square inch.

Mutate - A change in the nucleus of a cell that differs from the original cell and constitutes a new variety of cell.

Mutation – A change or alteration in the gradual evolution of a microorganism.

Mycology – The study of molds, yeasts, and fungi.

Myelogram - An injection of a contrast medium (radiopaque dye) into the spinal cord to take an x-ray picture.

Myocardial infarction (MI) - The death of heart muscle from the sudden blockage of a coronary artery by a blood clot; also called heart attack.

Myocardium - Middle layer of the heart wall; heart muscle.

Mμ – Millimicron (nanometer).

μ – Micron.

μg – Microgram.

μl – Microliter.

μm – Micrometer, micron.

μmol – Micromole.

μOsm – Micro-osmole.

N

N – Nitrogen.

N - Normal (strength of solution).

Na – Sodium.

NaCl – Sodium chloride.

Nasal - Pertaining to the nose.

Nasal cannula - A device used for oxygen administration via the nose.

Nasal catheter - A catheter with side openings and an open end tip used for administration of oxygen via the nose.

Nasal packing - Material used for packing the nose to stop nasal hemorrhaging.

Nasogastric (NG) - Referring to the passage from the nose to the stomach.

Nasogastric tube (NGT) - A tube that passes through the patient's nose and throat and ends in the patient's stomach that allows for direct tube feeding to maintain the nutritional status of the patient or removal of stomach acids.

Nasopharynx – The portion of the pharynx above the palate.

Nasoplasty – A cosmetic surgery procedure performed to change the shape of the nose to create a more pleasing appearance; can be performed at the same time as a functional (reconstructive surgery) procedure such as a septoplasty to improve breathing difficulties; also called rhinoplasty.

Natal - Pertaining to birth.

National Fire Protection Association (NFPA) – A voluntary organization that develops international standards to reduce the incidence of fire and other hazards; sets standards for fire burden for all disposable packaged items stored and used within healthcare facilities and the fire standards for patient drapes used in the operating room.

National Patient Safety Goals (The Joint Commission) – An initiative established to help accredited organizations address specific areas of concern regarding patient safety.

Natural immunity - Immunity with which a person or animal is born.

Nebulizer - A device used to administer medication to people in the form of a mist inhaled into the lungs.

Necropsy – A post-mortem examination or autopsy.

Necrosis - Death of a mass of tissue while part of the living body.

Needle - A slender, hollow instrument for introducing material into or removing material from the body; also used for puncturing or suturing.

Needle holder – A surgical instrument used to drive suture needles to close or rejoin a wound or surgical site.

Negative air pressure – The situation that occurs when air flows into a room or area because the pressure in the area is less than that of surrounding areas.

Negative variance (accounting) – An undesirable difference in dollars and/or percents between expected costs forecasted in the departmental operating budget and actual costs determined by the facility's record keeping and accounting system.

Negotiation – A process in which parties with mutual interests reach agreement about disputes, determine courses of action, and bargain as necessary for their individual and mutual advantage.

Neonatal - Concerning the newborn.

Neoplasm - Abnormal growth of cells; tumor.

Nephrectomy – Surgical procedure to remove the kidney.

Radical nephrectomy removes the kidney, the adrenal gland, nearby lymph nodes, and other surrounding tissue. Simple nephrectomy removes just the affected kidney. Partial nephrectomy removes the tumor, but not the entire kidney.

Nephron - Microscopic functional unit of the kidney.

Nerve - Nerve fibers outside the central nervous system.

Net price – The total or per unit amount paid for something after all discounts have been applied to the purchase price.

Netiquette – Internet rules of workplace conduct that include respecting privacy guidelines and refraining from visiting offensive or illegal websites.

Network (personal interaction) – Formal and informal groups of persons with whom one communicates and interacts.

Network (technology) – A configuration of computers that enables users to share data, programs, and devices such as printers.

Neuritis - Inflammation of a nerve.

Neurologist - A doctor specializing in the treatment and diagnosis of disease of, or injury to, the nervous system.

Neurology - The branch of medicine that deals with the diagnosis and treatment of disorders or disease of the nervous system.

Neuron - Nerve cell.

Neutral - Neither acid nor base.

Neutralizer - Substance added to a medium which stops the action of a antimicrobial agent.

Newborn intensive care unit (NICU) - An intensive care unit designed for premature and ill newborn babies; also called neonatal intensive care unit.

NFPA - National Fire Protection Association.

ng – Nanogram (millimicrogram).

NG – Nasogastric.

NGT – Nasogastric tube.

NIA – Nursing information system.

NIBP - Non-invasive blood pressure.

NICU - Newborn intensive care unit.

Nipple shield - Cover worn over a nursing breast to protect the natural nipple.

nm – Nanometer (millimicron).

NMC – Nurse management council.

Node – A small mass of tissue such as a lymph node; space between cells in the myelin sheath.

Noise (communication) – Influences on communication that impact the interpretation and understanding of the message being communicated.

Nomenclature – A system of names used to identify parts of a mechanism or device.

Non-critical items (Spaulding classification system) – Items that contact intact skin.

Non-critical zone – An area of a gown or drape where direct contact with blood, body fluids, and other potentially infectious materials is unlikely to occur.

Non-exempt employees (Fair Labor Standards Act) – Employees who are not covered by requirements of the Fair Labor Standards Act; generally those who are salaried and earning more than a specific minimum who perform executive-type duties that include supervisory and management responsibilities.

Non-invasive blood pressure (NIBP) – The use of oscillometric equipment that uses a calibrated electronic device with a numerical readout of blood pressure to detect blood flow.

Nonionic - Atoms with no electrical charges; compounds containing a nondissociated hydrophilic group which forms a bond with water.

Nonlipid virus - A virus whose nucleic acid core is not surrounded by a lipid envelope. These viruses are generally more resistant to inactivation by disinfectants.

Nonpathogenic - Not capable of producing disease.

Nonpyrogenic - Free from fever-causing substances.

Non-rebreathing circuit - An anesthesia breathing circuit which includes a reservoir bag, wide-bore corrugated tubing, and a spring-loaded expiratory valve. This system is semi-closed to prevent rebreathing by having the gas flow rate from the cylinders slightly in excess of the patient's minute respiratory volume.

Nontoxic - Not poisonous; not capable of producing injury or disease.

Non-verbal communication – The process of communication by sending and receiving wordless messages; also called body language.

Nonwoven - Fabric made by bonding (as opposed to weaving) fibers together.

Normal flora - Normal bacterial population of a given area.

Nose - Nasal cavity.

Nosocomial – Hospital-acquired infection (HAI); relates to a disease acquired as a result of treatment in a hospital.

NPO – Nothing by mouth.

NS—Normal saline.

NSR—Nasal sinus reconstruction.

Nuclear medicine - Specialty dealing with moderate amounts of radioactive materials used in diagnostic procedures in radiology.

Nucleotide - Building block of deoxyribonucleic acid (DNA) and ribonucleic acid (RNA).

Nucleus - Functional center of a cell that governs activity and heredity.

Nurse – A professional skilled or trained in the caring for the sick.

Nurse anesthetist - A registered nurse with additional

training in anesthesia.

Nursing information system (NIS) – A computer-based system that manages clinical data from a variety of healthcare environments and provides necessary information in a timely and orderly manner to help nurses improve patient care.

O

Oath (legal) – Swearing to tell the truth, the whole truth, and nothing but the truth.

OB pads - Extra-long sanitary pads used to absorb vaginal flow following the birth of a child.

OB-GYN – Obstetrics and gynecology

Objection (legal) – A request that the court (judge) not allow a question to be asked of a witness by an opposing lawyer because it is illegal, confusing, or improper.

Obstetrician - A doctor who practices obstetrics.

Obstetrics - The branch of medicine that deals with pregnancy and childbirth.

Occlude - To close or bring together.

Occupancy (safety) – The number of persons that can legally be present in a building or room at the same time.

Occupational Safety and Health Administration (OSHA) – A federal government agency organized within the U.S. Department of Labor that is concerned with a safe work environment and employee safety.

Occurrence Report (confidential) – A written report of an unusual unplanned incident involving patient safety.

Ocular - Of the eye; eyepiece of an optical instrument.

Offer – A proposal to perform an act or to pay an amount that, if accepted, constitutes a legally valid contract.

Ohm - Unit of measurement that expresses the amount of resistance to the flow of an electric current.

Olfactory - Pertaining to the sense of smell.

On-boarding – The process of welcoming and integrating new employees into their work environment.

On-budget – A financial term meaning that actual expenditures are in line with budgeted (expected) expenditures.

On call – Employee standby status where employees are ready to be called into work if needed.

Oncology - Study of tumors.

Oophorectomy - The removal of one or both ovaries.

Opened but unused – A single-use disposable device whose sterility has been breached or compromised or whose sterile package was opened even though the device had not been used on a patient or been in contact with blood or body fluids.

Open-ended (question) – A question that permits applicants to respond in an unstructured way and that is used to ask for opinions and ideas requiring more than just a few words.

Open reduction internal fixation (ORIF) – A method to surgically repair a fractured bone by using plates and screws or an intramedullary (IM) rod to stabilize the bone.

Operating budget (departmental) – A detailed plan for generating revenue, if any, and managing expenses to meet Central Service financial goals; also called budget or expense budget.

Operating suite - A room in the surgery department designed for performing a surgical procedure.

Operation - A procedure performed on a living body.

Ophthalmic - Pertaining to the eye.

Ophthalmology - The branch of medicine concerned with the study of the physiology, anatomy, and pathology of the eye and the diagnosis and treatment of disorders of the eye.

Ophthalmoscope - A device used to examine the retina and interior structures of the eye; includes a mirror that reflects light into the eye and a central hole through which the eye is examined.

Opportunists - Microbes that produce infection only under especially favorable conditions.

Opportunity cost – The cost of passing up the next best choice when making a decision. Example: if product A is purchased, opportunity cost is the value of the next best purpose for which the money could be used.

Optical scanning – The process of using a computer input device to scan information from bar codes directly into a computer system; see bar code.

Optimum temperature (bacterial growth) - The temperature at which bacteria grow best.

Oral and maxillofacial surgery - Surgery to correct a wide spectrum of diseases, injuries and defects in the head, neck, face, jaws and the hard and soft tissues of the oral and maxillofacial region.

Oral hygiene swab - Treated applicator used to clean the mouth.

Oral reprimand – A documented spoken warning to an employee to correct inappropriate behavior.

Oral suction catheter – A hollow tube used to aspirate oral and nasal cavities.

Oral suction machine - A device used to suction liquids and mucus from the oral and nasal cavities.

Orchiectomy - Surgery to remove the testicles.

Order (product or service) – The process by which a buyer makes specific commitments to a seller or service provider relating to a specific purchase.

Order point (order quantity system) – A method of reordering a predetermined quantity of products when a predetermined on-hand level is reached.

Organ – A part of the body containing two or more tissues that function together for a specific purpose.

Organic - Compounds containing oxygen, carbon and hydrogen; characteristic of, pertaining to, or derived from living organisms.

Organism – A living thing, plant or animal; may be unicellular or multicellular.

Organization chart – A graphic usually presented as a flow outline that identifies position titles and relationships in an organization.

Organizational culture – A set of understandings shared by members of an organization that are relevant and distinctive, that are passed on to new members, and that influence organizational decision-making.

Orientation – The process of providing basic information about a healthcare facility that must be known by employees in all departments.

Orientation checklist – A document that identifies topics to be addressed in the orientation process; when completed, it provides a record that verifies the information provided to the employee.

ORIF – Open reduction internal fixation

Origin - Source; beginning; end of a muscle attached to a non-moving part.

Orthopedic felt - Material used for a cushioning effect under casts and splints.

Orthopedics – A specialty concerned with the correction or prevention of skeletal deformities.

ORYX® (The Joint Commission) – An initiative that integrates outcomes and other performance measurement data into The Joint Commission's accreditation process.

OSHA - Occupational Safety and Health Administration.

Osmosis - Net movement of solvent molecules across a selectively permeable membrane from areas of higher to lower concentrations.

Osmotic pressure - Tendency of a solution to draw water into it; directly related to the concentration of the solution.

Ossification – The process by which cartilage is replaced by bone.

Osteoblast - Bone-forming cell.

Osteomyelitis - Inflammation of bone marrow.

Osteoporosis - Abnormal loss of bone tissue with tendency to fracture.

Osteotome - Chisel-like instrument used to cut or shave bone.

Ostomy - An operation to create an opening from an area inside the body to the outside. See Colostomy.

OTC – Over the counter; a drug that can be obtained without a prescription.

Otitis media - Inflammation of the middle ear.

Otoscope - A hand-held instrument which includes a magnification lens and light used to examine the ear canal and eardrum; an ear speculum (a funnel shaped attachment) is attached to allow the physician to direct the light at a particular point; also called auriscope.

Outcome – A healthcare quality indicator that assesses the extent to which healthcare services have improved or maintained a patient's health.

Outpatient care services – Services provided by a hospital to patients who are not admitted to the facility.

Outpatient Surgery Services – A unit within a hospital's Surgical Services division that provides surgical services for patients not requiring admittance to the facility; also called same day surgery (SDS) or ambulatory services.

Outsource – The act of purchasing a product or service from an external provider that could, alternatively, be provided by the facility's own employees.

Outsourcing (equipment) - Transfer of control of a hospital's equipment management system to an external entity.

Ovaries - Female reproductive glands.

Overstock – An excessive amount of a product in storage.

Overtime (budget standard) – The number of labor hours worked in excess of the number of labor hours that are scheduled.

Ovulation - Release of a mature ovum from a follicle in the ovary.

Ovum - Female sex cell.

Oxidation – The process by which a molecule, atom, or ion loses an electron; act or process of oxidizing: chemical breakdown of nutrients for energy.

Oxidative chemistries – A class of compounds containing an additional atom of oxygen bound to oxygen that uses oxidation to interrupt cell function.

Oxidize - To change by increasing the proportion of the electronegative part or change (an element or ion) from a lower to higher positive valence.

Oxidizing agent - Material that removes electrons from another substance.

Oximeter - A device that monitors the amount of oxygen carried by the hemoglobin in red blood cells. In bloodless medicine, any blood a patient loses is not replaced by transfusion, so it is extremely important to monitor how much oxygen the patient's body is receiving from the remaining blood.

Oxygen - Gas needed to completely break down nutrients for energy within the cell.

Oxygenator - Device which mechanically oxygenates venous blood extracorporeally. They are used in combination with one or more pumps for maintaining circulation during open heart surgery and for assisting the circulation in patients seriously ill with some cardiac and pulmonary disorders.

Oxygen mask – A covering used to facilitate the administration of oxygen.

Oxygen monitor - A medical equipment device that provides continuous oxygen monitoring for anesthesia delivery equipment as well as hospital and home ventilators.

Oxygen saturation - The ratio of oxygen volume carried by the blood to the potential oxygen-carrying capacity of the blood.

oz – Ounce.

Ozone - A reactive and unstable oxygen molecule.

P4P – Pay for performance.

PA - Peracetic acid.

Pacemaker - Any of several usually miniaturized and surgically implanted electronic devices used to stimulate or regulate contractions of the heart muscle.

Packaging - Application or use of appropriate closures, wrappings, cushioning, containers, and complete identification up to, but not including, the shipping container and associated packing.

$PaCO_2$ – Partial pressure of carbon dioxide in arterial blood.

Pallet – A portable platform (rack) used to store and/or move case goods of products that are stacked upon it.

Pancreas - A large fleshy gland located behind the stomach that secretes a digestive fluid and insulin.

Pancreatectomy - Surgery to remove the pancreas. In a total pancreatectomy, the duodenum, common bile duct, gallbladder, spleen, and nearby lymph nodes also are removed.

Pandemic – A very widespread epidemic, even of worldwide extent.

PaO_2 – Partial pressure of oxygen in arterial blood.

PAP – Papanicolaou smear.

Papanicolaou smear (PAP) – A screening test for early detection of cervical cancer.

Paper trail – Written evidence or records that document an activity, process, or event.

Papers (kraft-type) - Medical grade paper packaging material used for numerous sterilization applications.

Paperwork – A slang term referring to forms, applications, and/or other written documents that must be completed, for example, by a new employee beginning work at a healthcare facility.

PAR - Periodic automatic replenishment of inventory.

Par cart – A distribution method in which a supply cart remains in a given location and is inventoried and replenished on a regular basis.

Par level (inventory) – The desired amount of inventory which should be on hand.

Paracentesis – A puncture through the wall of a cavity, usually to remove fluid or promote drainage.

Paramedic – A person with a professional certification who works in the health care field in an annually capacity who primarily provides pre-hospital advanced medical care.

Parametric release - Declaring a product to be sterile on the basis of physical and/or chemical process data rather than on the basis of sample testing or biological indicator results.

Paraplegia - Paralysis of the legs and sometimes the lower part of the body, usually caused by an injury to the spinal cord.

Parasite – A plant or animal that lives upon or within another living organism (host) from which it obtains nourishment and at whose expense it grows without giving anything in return.

Parenteral - Denoting any route for introducing substances other than the alimentary canal.

Parenteral hyperalimentation - Intravenous administration of total nutrient requirements through a central venous catheter.

Parenteral solutions - Solutions administered to patients intravenously.

Parietal - Pertaining to the wall of a space or cavity.

Particle – A piece of matter with observable length, width, and thickness; usually measured in microns.

Particulate matter – The general term applied to matter of miniature size with observable length, width, and thickness contrasted to non-particulate matter without definite dimension.

Partnership – A relationship between parties that involves a mutual goal and defined responsibilities.

Parturition - Childbirth; labor.

PARU - Post-anesthesia recovery unit; also known as PACU or Post Anesthesia Care Unit.

Passivation – A chemical process applied during instrument manufacture that provides a corrosion-resistant finish by forming a thin and transparent oxide film.

Passive carrier – A carrier who harbors the causative agent of a disease without having had the disease.

Passive immunity - Immunity produced without the body of the person or animal that becomes immune participating in its production; example: production of immunity to diphtheria by injection of diphtheria antitoxin.

Pasteurization – The process of heating a fluid to a moderate temperature for a definite period of time to destroy undesirable bacteria without changing its chemical composition.

Patella - Kneecap.

Pathogen - Capable of causing disease; disease-producing microorganism.

Pathogenic - Capable of producing disease.

Pathologist - A physician especially trained in the cause and nature of disease.

Pathology - Study of disease.

Patient care equipment - Portable (mobile) equipment used to assist in the care and treatment of patients; examples: suction units and heat therapy units.

Patient care services department – A department that involves direct contact with patients and provides medical care to them.

Patient-controlled analgesia (PCA) - Provides for automatic administration of pain medication.

Patient days – A unit in a system of accounting used by health care facilities and health care planners. Each day represents a unit of time during which the services of the institution or facility are used by a patient. For example, 50 patients in a hospital for 1 day would represent 50 patient days.

Patient days (adjusted) – An adjustment factor for admissions and patient days to reflect the volume of outpatient activity and its impact.

Pawl – A pivoted tongue or sliding bolt on one part of an instrument adapted to fall into notches or interdental space on another part to permit motion in only one direction.

Pay for performance (Medicare) – An initiative to encourage improved quality of care in which Medicare beneficiaries receive healthcare services that involve collaboration with healthcare providers and other stakeholders. Its aims are to ensure use of valued quality measures, that providers are not in conflict, and that they have support for achieving actual improvement; abbreviated "P4P."

p.c. – After meals.

PCA - Patient-controlled analgesia.

PCD – Process challenge device.

PCU - Progressive care unit. For patients who do not need intensive care, but who do need more nursing care than what is usually provided on general nursing units.

PDA – Personal digital assistant.

PDCA – Plan-do-check-act.

Pediatrics - A branch of medicine dealing with the development, care, and disease of children.

Peds – Pediatrics.

Peel pouch – paper sterilization enclosure with a clear plastic side designed to contain single items readily visible to the user.

PEL - Permissible exposure limits

Pelvic inflammatory disease (PID) - A general term that refers to infection of the uterus (womb), fallopian tubes, and other reproductive organs.

Pelvic sling - A device that supports the pelvis.

Pelvis - Basin-like structure; lower portion of the abdomen; large bone of the hip.

Pelvis traction - Traction applied to the back with a belt that encircles a patient's waist with weights attached.

Penicillin - Antibiotic produced by the mold, Penicillium notatum.

Penile implant - Surgical insertion of a prosthesis to enable the patient to obtain an erection.

Penis - Male organ of urination and intercourse.

Peracetic acid (PA) - Liquid oxidizing agent that is an effective biocide at low temperatures; used in a sterilization system that processes immersible diagnostic and surgical instruments (primarily flexible and rigid scopes); items must be used immediately after sterilization because they are wet and cannot be stored.

Percutaneous transluminal coronary angioplasty (PTCA) – A surgical procedure performed to open blocked coronary arteries caused by coronary artery disease (CAD) and to restore arterial blood flow to the heart tissue without open-heart surgery.

Performance appraisal – An objective and comprehensive employee rating or evaluation.

Performance counseling – Activities to improve performance and productivity by providing an employee with feedback about strengths and where improvement is required; see performance improvement plan.

Performance improvement (patients) - A process to continually improve patient care that identifies performance functions and associated costs which affect patient outcomes and the perception of patients and families about the quality and value of services provided.

Performance improvement plan (employees) – A plan resulting from performance counseling designed to provide employees with constructive feedback about specific areas where improvement is needed and steps to attain performance goals.

Performance management – The process of maintaining or improving employee job performance with performance assessment tools, coaching and counseling, and providing on-going feedback.

Performance qualification (PQ) - Obtaining and documenting evidence that equipment, as installed and operated in accordance with operational procedures, consistently performs according to predetermined factors and meets specifications.

Performance standards – Task requirements that are employee goals.

Perfusion: The process of flooding fluid through the artery to saturate the surrounding tissue.

Peri pad – A mass of material used to absorb vaginal flow.

Pericardial - Area between the heart and the sac enveloping the heart.

Perineal prostatectomy- Surgery to remove the prostate through an incision made between the scrotum and the anus.

Perineum - Pelvic floor; external region between the anus and genital organs.

Periodic automatic replenishment (PAR) - Inventory system in which the desired amount of products which should be on hand is established, and inventory replenishment returns the quantity of products to this level; also called par system.

Periosteum – The membrane of connective tissue that closely invests all bones except at the articular surface.

Peripheral - Located away from a center or central structure.

Peripheral device – Electronic equipment such as a printer or scanner that is connected to a computer.

Peripheral edema – The build-up of fluid in the ankles, feet, and legs.

Peripheral nervous system - All nerves and nerve tissue outside the central nervous system.

Peristalsis – Wave-like movements in the wall of an organ or duct that propel its contents forward.

Peritoneum – A serous membrane that lines the abdominal cavity, forms the outer layer of abdominal organs, and forms supporting ligaments for some organs.

Peritonitis - Inflammation of the peritoneum.

Permissible exposure limits (PEL) - Limits developed by the Occupational Safety and Health Administration to indicate the maximum airborne concentration of a contaminant to which an employee may be exposed over the duration specified by the type of PEL assigned to that contaminant.

Perpetual inventory system – A system that tracks all incoming and issued supplies to determine, on an on-going basis, the quantity of supplies in storage.

PERRLA – Pupils equal, round, react to light and accommodation

Personal digital assistant (PDA) – A mobile hand-held computer that stores and displays information and functions as a cellular phone, fax sender, web browser, and personal organizer.

Personal protective equipment (PPE) – Specialized clothing or equipment worn by an employee for protection against a hazard.

Personnel budget – A budget that forecasts labor costs for a specific time period. It includes all compensation applicable to Central Service personnel including salaries, wages, and benefits; also called labor budget or compensation budget.

Personnel records – All information about individual employees that is collected and maintained by the employer. Human resources personnel may monitor primary documents, but Central Service departments may maintain training and other department-specific documentation.

Pertussis - Whopping cough.

Petri dish - A shallow, covered cylindrical glass or plastic dish used to culture bacteria and in which bacterial colonies may be observed without removing the cover.

Pezzer catheter - A device with a particular retaining mechanism used for urinary suprapubic drainage and drainage of body cavities.

Phagocyte - Cell capable of ingesting bacteria or other foreign particles.

Phagotization – The process by which some cells can ingest bacteria or other foreign particles.

Phalanges - Bones that comprise the fingers and toes.

Pharynx - Throat.

Phased retirement – A work schedule allowing employees near retirement to gradually reduce their work hours over a period of time.

Phenol - Carbolic acid (phenyl alcohol); a colorless crystalline compound with strong disinfectant properties.

Phenol coefficient – A method of designating the disinfecting properties of a chemical by comparing its activity to that of phenol.

Phlebitis - Inflammation of a vein.

Phlebotomist - A health professional trained to draw blood.

Phlebotomy - Entry into a vein with a needle for the purpose of letting blood out of the body.

Physical ability test – A test that determines an individual's ability to perform job functions or tasks when physical strength or endurance is required.

Physical examination (work-related) – A medical examination performed to determine if an individual can perform the physical requirements of a job.

Physical monitors – Time, temperature, and pressure recorders, displays, digital printouts, and gauges used to assure that all sterilization parameters have been met.

Physical therapy - Treatment of injury and disease by mechanical or physical means such as exercise, heat, light, and massage.

Physiology - Study of the function of living organisms.

PI – Performance improvement

Pick and pack – An inventory control system for forms and office supplies. Items are shipped/charged to the customer as ordered in minimal quantities, and the customer is financially responsible for the vendor's agreed-upon inventory.

PID – Pelvic inflammatory disease.

Pilferage – The act of stealing small quantities over a relatively long time period.

Pink slip – A slang term referring to a written notice given to employees being terminated or laid-off.

Pipette - A glass or transparent plastic tube used to measure and transfer small quantities of liquid.

Piston syringe - Instrument used for irrigation.

PKU – Phenylketonuria.

Placenta – The structure that nourishes and maintains the developing individual during pregnancy.

Plague – An acute, often fatal epidemic disease caused by Pasteurella pestis and transmitted to man by fleas from rats and other rodents.

Plaintiff – A person who brings an action in a court of law.

Plan-do-check-act (PDCA) – A quality process improvement technique that utilizes a sequential cycle (plan-do-check-act) to move toward a defect-free work system.

Plasma - The liquid portion of blood.

Plasmolysis - Shrinkage of a cell or its contents due to withdrawal of water by osmosis.

Plasmoptysis - Escape of protoplasm from a cell due to rupture of the cell wall.

Platelet – A cell fragment that forms a plug to stop bleeding and acts in blood clotting; thrombocyte.

Pleading claim (legal) – The act of preparing and presenting legal documents and arguments.

Pleura - Serous membrane that lines the chest cavity and covers the lungs.

PM – Preventive maintenance.

PMA – Pre-market approval.

PMS – Premenstrual syndrome.

Pneumatic tube (transport system) – A transport system built into a building's infrastructure that allows small, lightweight items such as papers to be moved between locations in plastic carriers that travel through tubes.

Pneumonectomy - An operation to remove an entire lung.

Pneumonia - Inflammatory consolidation or solidification of lung tissue due to presence of an exudate blotting out the air-containing spaces; see exudate.

Pneumothorax - Accumulation of air in the pleural space.

PO – By mouth.

PO_2 – Partial pressure of oxygen.

POD - Proof of delivery.

Point of use processing - That which occurs when a medical device is processed immediately before use and/or close to the patient care area.

Policy – A predetermined course of action that identifies a key activity and provides a general strategy; a written statement of intent.

Poliomyelitis – A viral disease in which there is inflammation of the gray substance of the spinal cord; commonly called infantile paralysis.

Pollution - State of rendering unclean or impure by adding harmful substances.

Polycarbonate – A type of plastic.

Polyethylene – A thermoplastic polymer capable of being produced in thin sheets; exhibits good moisture-vapor barrier qualities but has a high sloughing tendency.

Polymerize – The process of joining many simple molecules into long chains of more complex molecules whose molecular weight is a multiple of the original and whose physical properties are different.

Polyp – A protruding growth (often grape-like) from a mucous membrane.

Polypropylene – A type of plastic.

Polystyrene – A type of plastic.

Polyurethane – A type of plastic.

Polyvinyl chloride (PVC) – A type of plastic.

Porous - Possessing or full of pores (minute openings).

Portability - Not fixed; can be transported.

Portable suction unit – A mechanical suction device powered by battery or electrical current and used in various facility locations.

Portal of entry (chain of infection) - Path by which an infectious agent enters a susceptible host.

Portal of exit (chain of infection) - Path by which an infectious agent leaves the reservoir.

Position control – A process that imposes restrictions on filling vacant positions to manage the costs associated with them.

Positive air pressure – The situation in which air flows out of a room or area because the pressure in the area is greater than that of surrounding areas.

Positive discipline – Any action to encourage proper behavior; also called positive reinforcement or positive feedback.

Poss - Possible.

Post-Anesthesia Care Unit (PACU) – A unit within the Operating Room Department where patients recover from anesthesia under close supervision; also called Post-Anesthesia Recovery Unit (PARU).

Post-anesthesia recovery unit (PARU) – See post-anesthesia care unit.

Posterior repair - The repair of a rectocele, a herniation of the rectum into the vagina, which can occur if the pelvic muscles are weakened by childbirth.

Posterior - Toward the back; dorsal.

Postnasal balloon - A device used to stop nasal hemorrhaging.

Postnatal - Occurring after birth.

Pounds per square inch gauge (psig) – A measure of ambient air pressure; the pressure that a gas would exert on the walls of a one-cubic foot container.

Power sources- Devices that supply energy; for example batteries or compressed air for powered surgical instruments.

PPD – Purified protein derivative (of tuberculin).

PPE - Personal protective equipment.

PPM – Parts per million.

PQ - Performance qualification.

Preconditioning – The treatment of a product prior to the sterilization cycle in a room or chamber to attain specified limits for temperature and relative humidity; see conditioning.

Preconditioning area – The chamber or room in which preconditioning occurs.

Prefix (word element) – The word element that comes before the root word element.

Preliminary Accreditation (The Joint Commission) – Results when the health care organization demonstrates compliance with selected standards in the surveys conducted under the Early Survey Policy.

Preliminary Denial of Accreditation (The Joint Commission) – Results when there is justification to deny accreditation as evidenced by an Immediate Threat to Health or Safety situation; or the organization failed to resolve the requirements of a Conditional Accreditation; or it was in significant noncompliance with The Joint Commission Standards.

Pre-market approval (PMA) – Approval granted to manufacturers of new devices by the Food and Drug Administration to demonstrate that the devices are safe and effective.

Pre-market notification application (510k) – A comprehensive package of information designed to demonstrate that the new product is substantially equivalent to one or more medical devices already being marketed.

Premenstrual syndrome (PMS) - A wide range of physical or emotional symptoms that typically occur 5 to 11 days before a woman starts her monthly menstrual cycle.

Prenatal - Occurring before birth.

Preparation area – A designated place for the assembling, wrapping, and packaging of articles, trays, and basins prior to sterilization.

Preservative – A substance that prevents biologic decomposition of materials when added to them.

Pressure gauge - A device for indicating pressure such as of the sterilizer jacket or chamber.

Preventive maintenance (PM) - Service provided to equipment to maintain it in proper operating condition by providing planned inspection, and by detecting and correcting failures before they occur.

Price quotation – A request made by a purchaser to a vendor for the current price of a product or service that meets the facility's quality requirements.

Primary infection – The first of two or more infections.

Prion – A disease-causing agent that is not bacterial, fungal, or viral and contains no genetic material. It is a protein that occurs normally in a harmless form but, by folding into an abnormal shape, the normal prion turns into a rogue agent. It then co-opts other normal prions to become rogue prions. Prions have been held responsible for a number of degenerative brain diseases, including scrapie (a fatal disease of sheep and goats), mad cow disease, Creutzfeldt-Jacob disease, and others.

Privileged information (legal) – Information learned in the context of a protected relationship such as between an attorney and client or a doctor and patient.

PRN – As needed; whenever necessary.

PRN employee – An employee who is hired with no guarantee of scheduled hours to supplement full-and part-time staff; from Latin ("pro re nata") meaning "as needed."

Prostheses - Artificial substitutes for body parts, and materials inserted into tissue for functional, cosmetic, or therapeutic purposes. Prostheses can be functional, as in the case of artificial arms and legs, or cosmetic, as in the case of an artificial eye.

Pro time – Prothrombin time.

Probation (eligibility) – A trial period when the employer determines a person's suitability and capability for a position.

Probation (discipline) – The requirement that an employee's performance or conduct be closely monitored for a specified time.

Probe - A slender instrument used for surgical exploration.

Procedure - A series of actions to accomplish a task; a step-by-step way of doing something.

Process – A specific course of action required to achieve a result; a process is comprised of a number of steps.

Process challenge device (PCD) – An object that simulates a predetermined set of conditions when used to test sterilizing agent(s).

Process equivalency - Documented evaluation that the same sterilization process can be delivered by two or more pieces of sterilization equipment.

Process flow map – A chart showing the path (flow) that instrument trays and/or durable medical equipment take as they cycle through their daily routine.

Process improvement – An activity to identify and resolve work task-related problems that yield poor quality; the strategy of finding solutions to eliminate the root causes of process performance problems.

Process indicators - Devices used with individual units (examples: packs or containers) to demonstrate that the unit has been exposed to the sterilization process and to distinguish between processed and unprocessed units.

Processes (work) - Series of work activities which produce a product or service.

Processing area – An area in which decontaminated, clean instruments and other medical and surgical supplies are inspected, assembled into sets and trays, and wrapped, packaged, or placed into container systems for sterilization; also called "preparation and packaging area" if part of Central Service and "pack room" if textile packs are assembled there.

Processing group – A collection of products or product families that can be sterilized in the same EtO sterilization process. All products within the group have been determined to present an equal or lesser challenge to the sterilization process; see product family.

Proctology - A branch of medicine dealing with the structure and disease of the anus.

Proctoscope - An endoscope used for dilating and examining the rectum.

Proctoscopy - An examination of the rectum and the lower end of the colon using a thin lighted instrument called a sigmoidoscope.

Proctosigmoidoscopy - An examination of the rectum and the lower part of the colon using a thin, lighted instrument called a sigmoidoscope.

Procurement – The process of acquiring and evaluating goods and services beginning with determining needs through product utilization, conclusion of contracted service, or until the end of the useful life of a capital equipment item.

Product adoption – The process of formally including a candidate product into an existing validated sterilization process.

Product evaluation – The process of reviewing commodity-type items including gloves and catheter trays to make purchase specification decisions.

Product family – A collection of products determined to be similar or equivalent for validation purposes.

Product integrity check – The act of examining a sterile package to insure it is intact and uncompromised before being dispensed for use.

Product substitution – The need to use a replacement product when a currently used and desired item is unavailable.

Product usage cycle – The steps through which a product flows from when it is removed from inventory until it is replaced in inventory and when applicable storage records are up-dated.

Productivity – The ratio of the quality and quantity of output to the amount of input such as labor hours required to generate the output.

Professional communication standards – The established norms (protocols) that establish how professionals communicate with other professionals.

Profit center – A department or unit within a healthcare facility that generates revenue and to which applicable expenses are allocated so profitability can be determined.

Progesterone – The hormone produced by the corpus luteum and placenta; maintains the lining of the uterus for pregnancy.

Prognosis - Prediction of the probable outcome of a disease based on the patient's condition.

Program budget – A budget designed to control an out-of-the-ordinary expense that will have a significant impact on the operating budget; also called special purpose budget.

Progressive discipline – A program designed to modify employee behavior through a series of increasingly serious punishments for unacceptable behavior.

Proof of delivery (POD) – A signed document such as delivery invoice, delivery note, or packing slip verifying that the purchaser has received the goods, and they are acceptable.

Prophylactic – An agent used to prevent infection or disease.

Prophylaxis - Prevention of disease.

Prostatectomy - An operation to remove part or all of the prostate.

Prostate gland - Organ that produces a fluid element in semen that stimulates the motility of sperm.

Prosthesis - Artificial replacement of a body part such as an arm or leg.

Protein - Complex combinations of amino acids containing hydrogen, nitrogen, carbon, oxygen and, usually sulfur and sometimes other elements; essential constituents of all living cells.

Prothrombin - Clotting factor; converted to thrombin during blood clotting.

Proton – A positively-charged particle in the nucleus of an atom.

Protoplasm – A thick mucous-like substance that is colorless and translucent that forms the biochemical basis of life found within the cell nucleus.

Protozoa - Single-celled animals with no cell wall or with one composed of chitin, some of which live as parasites in the blood or tissue fluids of humans and animals.

Protozoan – A one-celled animal-like microorganism of the sub-kingdom, Protozoa.

Provisional Accreditation (The Joint Commission) – Results when a health care organization fails to successfully address all requirements for improvement in an Evidence of Standards Compliance (ESC) within 45 or 60 days following the posting of the Accreditation Summary Findings Report; see also Evidence of Standards Compliance.

Proximal - Nearer to point of origin or to a reference point.

Prudent - Marked by wisdom or judiciousness; wise.

Pseudopodia - "False feet;" temporary protrusions of ectoplasm to provide locomotion.

PSI– Pounds per square inch.

PSIA - Pounds per square inch absolute.

PSIG – Pounds per square inch gauge.

Psychiatrist - A physician who specializes in psychiatry.

Psychiatry - The branch of medicine that deals with the study, treatment, and prevention of mental illness.

Psychologist - A social scientist who studies behavior and mental processes, generally in a research or clinical setting.

Psychomotor skills – Steps required to perform specific jobs.

Psychrophiles (bacteria) - Cold-loving bacteria whose optimum temperature for growth is 59°F-68°F (15°C-20°C) or below.

PT – Physical therapy.

PTCA – Percutaneous transluminal coronary angioplasty.

PTH – Parathyroid hormone.

Public relations – Communication or other activities designed to create a favorable public image.

Pulmonary - Pertaining to the lungs.

Pulse oximeter - A small device that uses a light sensor to help determine if a patient has enough oxygen.

Pulse – A wave of increased pressure in blood vessels produced by contraction of the heart.

Punch list – A list developed after substantial completion of a project to determine defective or incomplete work that still must be done; also called inspection list.

Pupil – The opening in the center of the eye through which light enters.

Purchase order – A document used by the healthcare facility to inform a vendor that a shipment of specified items should be delivered at agreed-upon prices.

Purchase unit – The standard size of the package or container in which a product is typically purchased. Example: case of 25 boxes of latex-free gloves with 100 gloves per box.

Purchasing – The process of "buying:" placing an order, receiving a product or service, and paying the vendor.

Purchasing agent – A staff member in a large healthcare facility with responsibilities to purchase specific lines of products, services, supplies, or equipment; also called buyer.

Purchasing director – The top-level manager in a large healthcare facility with responsibilities for that organization's procurement function; also called purchasing manager.

Purchasing handbook – A document developed by the healthcare facility to inform vendors about the organization's purchasing policies and procedures that must be followed at all times.

Purchasing system (centralized) – A purchasing system in which all (or most) purchases are made by a designated purchasing agent or purchasing department.

Purchasing system (decentralized) – A purchasing system in which all (or most) purchases needed by a department are made by department heads or someone within their department who is designated to do so.

Pure culture – A specific bacterial growth of only one species of microorganism.

Purulent - Containing pus.

Pus – A semi-fluid creamy product of inflammation consisting of blood cells (mainly white), bacteria, dead tissue cells, and serum.

PVC – Premature ventricular contraction.

PVC - Polyvinyl chloride.

Pyrogenic - Pus-producing.

Pyrex – A type of hard glass made from borosilicate which is alkaline free.

Pyrexia - Fever.

Pyrogen – A fever-producing substance.

Pyrogenic - Fever-producing; by-products of bacterial growth or metabolism.

Q

q – Every.

q.d. – Every day.

q.h. – Every hour.

q.i.d. – Four times a day.

q2h – Every 2 hours.

Quadrant - One part of four; to be divided into four equal parts.

Quadriplegia - Paralysis that affects all four limbs.

Qualification testing (sterilizer) – Special monitoring required after sterilizer installation, relocation, malfunction, process failure, repair, and after utility repair.

Qualified personnel – Persons who are prepared by training and experience to perform a specified task.

Quality (product) – Suitability for intended use or purpose; the closer that an item comes to being suitable for its intended use, or that a service fulfills its intended purpose, the more appropriate is the quality of the product or service.

Quality (management) – The consistent delivery of products and services according to established standards.

Quality assurance - Comprehensive and measured efforts to provide total quality.

Quality circle – A skilled team of employees that meets regularly to identify quality issues, use specific techniques for analyzing and resolving problems, and make improvement recommendations.

Quality control – A statistical sampling method that measures production quality.

Quality improvement (QI) – The process of measuring the current output of a process and then modifying it to enhance outcomes, increase productivity, and/or decrease costs.

Quarantine - Isolation of infected persons and contacts who have been exposed to communicable diseases for the time equal to the longest incubation period of the disease to which they have been exposed; also, the holding of sterilized instrumentation, before being released for use, while biological indicators are examined to allow safe release of instruments for surgical procedures.

Quaternary compound – A group of disinfectants having derivatives of benzalkonium chloride as the active ingredient.

Quats - Quaternary; relating to organic compounds in which the central atom is attached to four functional groups; i.e., quaternary ammonium compounds.

Quiescent - Not active.

R

Rachet – See ratchet.

Radical cystectomy - Surgery to remove the bladder as well as nearby tissues and organs.

Radical prostatectomy - Surgery to remove the entire prostate. The two types of radical prostatectomy are retropubic prostatectomy and perineal prostatectomy.

Radiant warmer - A medical apparatus that consists of an open bed with an overhead warmer and is used to keep an infant warm; also called infant warmer.

Radiation heat - Transmission of heat from one object to another without heating the space in between; the process of emitting radiant energy in the form of waves or particles.

Radio frequency identification (RFID) - A system in which the identity (serial number) of an item is wirelessly transmitted with radio waves.

Radiologist - A physician specializing in the use of radiant energy for diagnostic and therapeutic purposes.

Radiology - The science of radioactive substances and high-energy radiations.

Radiolucent - The property of relative transparency to the passage of X-rays through a material; example: a radiolucent table permits the passage of x-rays without leaving a shadow on the film. Soft tissues are radiolucent; bones are not.

Radiopaque - Being impenetrable to various forms of radiation.

Radiotherapy - The treatment of disease by means of x-rays or radioactive substances.

Radius - One of the two bones in the forearm.

Random numbers (table) – A compilation of numbers generated in an unpredictable, haphazardous sequence used to create a random sample.

Random sampling – A survey tactic in which, for example, each instrument set or case cart being analyzed for quality has an equal chance of being selected for analysis.

Range of motion - joint (ROM) – Joint flexibility; usually measured by the number of degrees from the starting position of a segment to its position at the end of its full range of the movement.

Ratchet - Part of a surgical instrument that "locks" the handles in place.

Rationale - Underlying reason; basis.

RCA - Root cause analysis.

Reagent – A substance used in laboratory analysis.

Reasonable accommodations (Americans with Disabilities Act) – Any change in the work environment or in the way things are customarily done that enables an individual with a disability to enjoy equal employment opportunities.

Reassignment – The process of transferring employees to alternative positions where their talents or skills may be best utilized for their own or the facility's benefit or where they can better perform the job according to required standards.

Rebate – An after-purchase discount offered by the maker or seller of a product; also called cash back offer.

Rebreathing circuit – A device used during the administration of anesthesia in which the exhaled gas is recirculated to the patient with CO_2 removed.

Recall – As in load recall, items to be returned to sterile processing because one or more indicators reveal that the load or items did not meet sterilization parameters. Also a manufacturer's recall of supplies or items suspected of not meeting production standards.

Receiver (communication) – A person who receives a message through a communication channel.

Receiving – The transfer of ownership from a vendor to a healthcare facility that occurs when products are delivered.

Recessive – A gene that is not expressed if a dominant gene for the same trait is present.

Reciprocal review – A performance appraisal method in which the employee and the manager evaluate each other based on agreed-upon factors.

Recommended Practices and Standards (AAMI) - Voluntary guidelines representing a consensus of AAMI members intended for use by healthcare facilities to help ensure the safety of medical instrumentation for patient use.

Recon – Reconstruction.

Reconstructive surgery - A surgical procedure performed to correct or repair abnormalities caused by injury, birth defects, disease, infections, or other surgeries; goal: to restore function and/or appearance to the body.

Recording graph - An apparatus designed for on-going graphical recording of the time, temperature, and duration of a sterilization cycle.

Record retention – The amount of time sterilization records are to be retained based upon each facility's risk management policy.

Rectal - Relating to the rectum; example: a rectal thermometer is an instrument that reads body temperature upon insertion in the rectum.

Rectum - The last several inches of the large intestine.

Redirect (legal) – Asking questions of one's own witness after cross-examination by the opposing lawyer; see "cross-examine."

Reduction mammoplasty – A (generally) outpatient procedure that involves the removal of fat, excess breast tissue, and skin and results in a smaller breast size; normally performed in women who are experiencing back pain or self-esteem issues; commonly called breast reduction.

Reflex – An involuntary response to a stimulus.

Refraction - Bending of light rays as they pass from one medium to another of a different density.

Regular full-time employee – An employee who works on a regular basis in the usual schedule of the facility's business for a specified number of weekly hours. Regular full-time employees are eligible for benefits.

Regular part-time employee – An employee who works on a regular basis in the usual schedule of the facility's business for a set amount of time weekly that is less than that worked by a full-time employee.

Regulation – A mandatory law or rule issued by a governing body.

Rel – Release.

Relative humidity – The amount of water vapor in the atmosphere; expressed as a percentage of the total amount of vapor the atmosphere could hold without condensation.

Rem – Remove.

Remedy – The means to attain justice in any matter in which legal rights are involved.

Remission – The diminution or abatement of disease symptoms.

Renal - Pertaining to the kidneys.

Re-order point – The number of purchase units that should be in inventory when an order is placed; see purchase unit.

Reorder point (ROP) - Inventory level available when an order is placed to replenish inventory.

Rep – Repair.

Repair (equipment) - Procedures used to return equipment to proper operating condition after it becomes inoperative.

Repetitive motion - Repeating the same movement(s) over and over again which could potentially cause injury.

Reprocessing - All of the steps performed to make a contaminated reusable or single-use device patient-ready; steps may include cleaning, functional testing, repackaging, relabeling, disinfection, or sterilization.

Request for information (RFI) – A process that collects information about potential vendors and their capabilities and develops strategies helpful in preparing a request for proposal; see request for proposal.

Request for proposal (RFP) – A request made by a purchaser to prospective vendors to learn the selling price of a product or service that meets identified quality requirements and other purchase concerns including quantity and timing of product delivery or service provision; also called Request for Quote (RFQ).

Requirement contracts – Commitments made by a purchaser to a vendor to purchase a minimum quantity of a specified product during a specific time period.

Requisition (non-stock) – An electronic or hardcopy document used to order something not held in inventory; for example; a preventive maintenance service.

Requisition (stock) – An electronic or hardcopy document used to request official inventory items from a storage area (issue requisition) or to be purchased (purchase requisition).

Requisition (traveling) – A requisition containing required ordering information completed by a department and routed to the purchasing department for order placement; used for repeat purchase of non-stock items used regularly but not stored in the department's storeroom.

Requisition system – A method of inventory distribution in which product needs are requested (requisitioned), and removed from a central storage location for transport to the user department.

Reservoir (carrier) – The carrier of an infectious microorganism; generally refers to a human carrier.

Reservoir of agent (chain of infection) – A place where an infectious agent (microorganism) can survive.

Resident bacteria - Bacteria normally occurring at a given anatomical site.

Residual (EtO) - Amount of EtO that remains inside materials after they are sterilized.

Residual (leftover) - Pertaining to or constituting what is remaining; leftover.

Residual property – The capacity of an antiseptic or disinfectant to kill microorganisms over a long period of time after initial application.

Resistance – The ability of an individual to ward off infection.

Resorption - Loss of substance (such as bone).

Resource – Something of value that is in limited supply and used to attain facility or departmental objectives; for example; people (labor hours), money, instruments, equipment, energy, and supplies.

Respiration – The exchange of oxygen and carbon dioxide between outside air and body cells.

Respirator - A device used to replace or assist breathing in a patient with respiratory problems.

Responsibility – One's obligation to achieve the goals and objectives associated with a specific position.

Resterilization - The application of a terminal process designed to remove or destroy all viable forms of microbial life, including bacterial spores, to an acceptable sterility assurance level; done for a device that has previously undergone a sterilization process.

Restraint - A device used to immobilize or hold back a patient.

Retina – The innermost layer of the eye; contains light sensitive cells (rods and cones).

Retinal detachment - Retinal detachment is a condition in which the sensory retina separates from the underlying pigment epithelium (surface). The detachment disrupts visual cell structure and thus markedly disturbs vision. Detachment is usually caused by a retinal tear and requires immediate surgical repair.

Retinoscope – An instrument used in retinoscopy that determines the refractive state of the eye. It provides a light source to illuminate the retina and then locates the aerial image of the retina in space to obtain an index of the refractive quality of the patient's lens system.

Retractors - Surgical instruments primarily used to move tissues and organs to keep them exposed throughout surgery.

Retroperitoneal - Behind the peritoneum (kidneys, pancreas, and abdominal aorta).

Retropubic prostatectomy - Surgical removal of the prostate through an incision in the abdomen.

Return on investment (ROI) – A ratio of the profit derived from a specific investment compared with its cost.

Reusable medical device – A device intended for repeated use on different patients with appropriate decontamination and other processing between uses.

Reusable surgical textile - Drape, gown, towel, or sterilization wrapper intended to be used during, or assist in preparing for surgery; made from a fabric (usually woven or knitted), fabric/film laminate, or non-woven material intended to be used more than once with appropriate reprocessing between uses.

Reuse - The repeated or multiple use of any medical device including those intended for single-use, with reprocessing (cleaning, disinfection, or sterilization) between uses.

Revenue – Money received by the healthcare facility or CSSD for products and services provided.

Revenue budget – A forecast of revenues that will be generated by or allocated to the CSSD during a specific time period.

Reverse osmosis – The diffusion (flowing) of water through a semi-permeable membrane to eliminate impurities; a water treatment process in which dissolved impurities are separated from water by forcing the water through a semi-permeable membrane under pressure.

RF – Rheumatic fever; rheumatoid factor.

RFI – Request for information.

RFID – Radio frequency identification.

RFP – Request for proposal.

Rh – Rhesus blood factor.

Rhinitis - Inflammation of the mucous membrane of the nose.

Rhinolaryngoscope - A rigid medical device used in the examination of the upper respiratory tract; includes a lamp at the tip for illumination and a built-in optical system.

Rhinoplasty - Plastic surgery performed to change the structure of the nose either to improve the appearance or to correct a deformity or injury; also called nose job.

Rib belt – A belt to provide compression of the thoracic area that may be used following surgery or rib fractures to resist expansion.

Rib spreaders – Retractors used to expose the chest.

Right-to-know – An Occupational Safety and Health Administration (OSHA) standard providing protection for workers from hazardous workplace substances by requiring employers to keep employees informed about hazardous substances they may handle.

Right-to-work – A state law that prohibits a requirement that an individual must join a union as a condition of employment.

Ringer's solution – A solution of sodium chloride, potassium chloride, and calcium chloride in water used for topical cleansing and irrigation.

Risk management – Methods to assess the risks of a specific activity and the subsequent development of a program to reduce exposure to these risks.

RLQ – Right lower quadrant.

Rm – Room.

RN – Registered nurse.

RNA – Ribonucleic acid.

Robinson catheter – A hollow tube used for urinary or wound drainage or aspiration.

Rod – A straight, slim mass of substance related to microorganisms; example: rod-shaped bacteria.

Role model – A person who serves as an example in a desired behavioral role within an organization.

Role play – A training exercise in which trainees pretend to be persons in situations addressed by the training who apply information presented in the training.

ROM – Range of motion (of joint).

Rongeur - Surgical instruments to cut or bite away at bone and tissue.

ROP – Reorder point.

Root (word element) – A word element that tells the primary meaning of a word; also called base word element.

Root cause – An identified reason for a problem or defect.

Root cause analysis (RCA) – A process that looks "backward" at an event to prevent its future occurrence.

Rubella - Measles.

Rumor – Information circulated without a source.

RUQ – Right upper quadrant.

Rx – Prescription.

S

Safety stock – The minimum amount of inventory that must be on hand.

SAL – Sterility assurance level.

Salary – Pay calculated on a weekly, monthly, or annual basis rather than at an hourly rate.

Salary range – A scale of pay rates from minimum to maximum established for a specific position.

Sales representatives – Persons selling products or services for a vendor or manufacturer. They often represent more than one product line from more than one company and usually work on commission; also called distributor sales representatives.

Salicylates - Aspirin and aspirin-related compounds.

Saline - Containing or pertaining to salt; an isotonic aqueous solution of sodium chloride for temporarily maintaining living cells.

Saliva - Secretion of salivary glands; moistens food and contains an enzyme that digests starch.

Salpingogram - An injection of a radiopaque dye into a fallopian tube to take an x-ray picture.

Salpingo-oophorectomy - Excision of a fallopian tube and ovary.

Salpingopexy - Surgical fixation of a fallopian tube.

Sanitary napkin - Material used during menstruation to absorb the uterine flow.

Sanitary - Relating to health; characterized by, or readily kept in, cleanness.

Sanitation - The promotion of hygiene and prevention of disease by maintenance of sanitary conditions.

Sanitize - To reduce the microbial flora in materials or on articles such as eating utensils to levels judged safe by public health standards.

Saponification – The action of detergent alkalis on an item's fat or soil contents to form soaps.

SAR – Statistical Analysis Report.

Sarcoma – A malignant tumor of connective tissue; a form of cancer.

Saturated – A condition that occurs when a chemical or liquid is added to a point where a substance can absorb no more.

Saturated steam - Steam that contains the maximum amount of water vapor; steam that exerts the maximum pressure for water vapor at a given temperature and pressure.

SBE – Subacute bacterial endocarditis.

Scalp vein needle - A device used to administer fluids via a vein.

Scalpel - A small, straight, thin-bladed knife used in surgery.

Scalpel blade - A razor-thin blade that adapts into the knife handle.

Scapula - Shoulder blade.

SCD - Sequential compression device.

Scissors - Surgical instruments used to cut, incise, and/or dissect tissue.

Sclera – The outermost layer of the eye; the "white" of the eye.

Scrotum – The sac in which the testes are suspended.

Scrubs – Uniform hospital attire worn by healthcare personnel.

Scrub tech – see surgical technologist.

SDS – Same day surgery.

Seals (tamper-evident) – A sealing method for sterile packaging that allows users to determine if packaging has been opened (contaminated) and helps them identify packages unsafe for patient use.

Search warrant – A court order issued by a judge or magistrate that authorizes an official to enter and search specified premises.

Sebaceous - Secreting or pertaining to sebum.

Sebum - An oily secretion of the sebaceous gland that lubricates the skin.

Sec – Second.

Secondary infection – A superimposed infection occurring in a host who is already suffering from an earlier infection.

Secretions - Substances produced by a gland.

Sedimentation - The process of solid particles settling at the bottom of a liquid.

Sedimentation rate - A common blood test used to detect and monitor inflammation in the body.

Selective action – The ability to inhibit or kill one group of microbes and not another.

Self-directed team – A multi-skilled group of empowered employees who share responsibility for producing and delivering a specific service or product.

Semen – A mixture of sperm cells and secretions from several male reproductive glands.

Semi-critical devices (Spaulding classification system) - Those that come in contact with non-intact skin or mucous membranes.

Seminal vesicle – The gland that produces semen.

Sender (communication) – A person who sends a message through a communication channel.

Seniority – Status determined by the length of time an employee has worked for a specific employer, department, or position within an organization.

Sensitivity - State of being susceptible.

Sensitization – The process of sensitizing or making susceptible.

Sentinel event (The Joint Commission) – An unexpected occurrence involving death or serious physical or psychological injury or the risk thereof.

Sentinel event policy (The Joint Commission) – An initiative designed to improve patient safety in all health care organizations that experience serious adverse events in patient care.

Sepsis – The condition, usually with fever, that results from the presence of microorganisms or their poisons in the blood stream or other tissues.

Septic - Relating to the presence of pathogens or their toxins.

Septicemia - Presence of pathogenic microorganisms or their toxins in the bloodstream; blood poisoning.

Septoplasty - A surgical procedure performed to correct nasal septum deviation: a failure of the nasal septum to be in the midline where it is supposed to be; done to improve the flow of air to the nose by repairing the malformed cartilage and/or the "bony" portion of the nose.

Septum - Dividing wall; examples: between heart chambers or sides of the nose.

Sequential compression device (SCD) - A device designed to limit the development of peripheral edema and deep vein thrombosis (DVT) in immobile patients; also called lymphedema pump.

Sequestering agents - Chemicals that remove or inactivate hard water minerals.

Sequestration - Removal or inactivation of water hardness elements by formation of a soluble complex or chelate.

Serious injury (Safe Medical Devices Act) – An injury or illness that is life-threatening; results in permanent impairment of a body function or permanent damage to body structure; or necessitates medical or surgical intervention to preclude permanent impairment of a body structure.

Serology - Science that deals with serum.

Serration - Parallel grooves in the jaws of surgical instruments.

Serum – A clear fluid exuded when blood coagulates.

Server – A computer that controls the flow of information along a network; see network.

Service – An activity that helps one or more persons or groups.

Service recovery – The sequence of steps to address customer complaints and problems to yield a win-win situation for the customer and the department.

Sexually transmitted disease (STD) - Venereal disease: a communicable infection transmitted by sexual intercourse or genital contact.

Sharps - Cutting instruments including knives, scalpels, blades, needles, scissors, chisels, osteotomes, some curettes, dissectors, elevators, rongeurs and cutting forceps, punches, saws and trocars.

Sheet wadding – A soft mass of material used for orthopedic padding.

Shelf life (disinfectants) – The length of time a disinfectant can be properly stored after which it must be discarded.

Shelf life (sterility) – The period of time during which product sterility is assumed to be maintained.

Shift differential – Additional compensation paid as an incentive for employees to work during a less-than-desirable work shift; examples: evening, weekend, and night shifts.

Shipping confirmation – A document sent by an equipment manufacturer to a distributor indicating that an equipment item has been shipped or is due to be shipped to the end user or the distributor's warehouse.

Shock – Life-threatening inadequate output of blood by the heart; also known as circulatory shock.

Short-term disability – A benefit that provides temporary income to an employee absent from the job for a period of time due to illness or injury.

Short-term exposure limit (STEL) - An employee's 15-minute time weighted average exposure which shall not be exceeded at any time during a work day unless another time period is specified by OSHA. If another time period is specified, the time weighted average exposure over that time period shall not be exceeded at any time during the working day;" see threshold limit value.

Shroud – A sheet or robe used to cover or protect a corpse.

SI – International System of Units .

SIADH – Syndrome of inappropriate antidiuretic hormone.

Sick leave – Paid time-off for employees who are out of work due to an illness or injury.

SIDS – Sudden infant death syndrome.

Sigmoid colon – The last portion of large intestine.

Sigmoidoscope - A thin, lighted tube-like instrument used to examine the inside of a colon.

Sigmoidoscopy - A minimally invasive medical examination of the large intestine from the rectum through the last part of the colon.

Sign - Manifestation of a disease noted by an observer.

Silicate - Mineral commonly in water derived from silica in quartz and other components.

Simple stain - Staining technique using only one dye.

Single sourcing – The concept of relying only on a single vendor as the source of one or more specific products.

Single-parameter indicator - Designed for one critical parameter that indicates exposure to a sterilization cycle at a stated value of the chosen parameter.

Single-use device (SUD) - A disposable item that is intended for use on one patient during a single procedure. It is not intended to be reprocessed (cleaned, disinfected, or sterilized) and used on another patient.

Situational leadership – A management style that recognizes there is no one best way to lead and that different situations and people require alternative leadership approaches.

Six sigma – A quality process that focuses on developing and delivering near-perfect products and services.

Skill set – The skills required to accomplish a specific task or function.

Skin graft – An excision of a flap of skin from one area of the body (donor site) to be transferred to another area.

Skin – The organ containing sweat glands that, through perspiration, produces and eliminates sweat.

Sling - A brace designed to give support to the arm and hand for bone and ligamentous injuries.

Sloughing - To cast off one's skin; to separate dead tissue from living tissue.

Sm – Small.

Small intestine – The digestive organ where the greatest amount of digestion and nutrient absorption into body cells occurs.

Smear – A thin layer of material spread on a glass slide for microscopic examination.

SMR—Submucosal resection.

SMS - Spunbond-meltblown-spunbond.

Soap – A compound of one or more fatty acids or their equivalent with an alkaline substance.

SOB – Short of breath.

Sodium – A major ingredient of extracellular fluids; plays a central role in the maintenance of the normal distribution of water in the body.

Sodium chloride 0.45 percent - An intravenous solution used for fluid and body electrolyte replacement.

Sodium chloride 5 percent - An intravenous solution used for fluid and body salt replacement.

Sodium chloride injection - A sterile, normal saline solution used to mix drug compounds for injections.

Sodium lactate - An intravenous solution used for fluid and electrolyte replacement.

Soft glass - Glass made from alkaline materials which cannot be subjected to high temperatures without causing chemical reactions and possible shredding of the glass.

Softening (sequestering) – The process of removing selected substances from hard water.

Soluble - Able to be dissolved.

Solute - A liquid, gas, or solid dissolved in a substance to make a solution.

Solution – A mixture with components evenly distributed.

Solvent – A liquid capable of dissolving another substance.

Sourcing (product) – Procedures used to determine the source from which products will be purchased.

Sourcing (vendor) – Activities undertaken to determine which, often from among many, vendors will be requested to quote prices for the products and services to be purchased by the healthcare facility.

sp gr – Specific gravity.

Span of control – A coordinating principle relating to the number of employees who can be supervised by one person.

Spaulding classification system – A system that classifies medical devices based on the degree of risk of infection.

spec – Specimen.

Special order – An order taken by a distributor for an item that is not available in the distributor's inventory and which must be ordered from the manufacturer.

Species - One kind of organism; the subdivision of a genus.

Specific gravity - A measure of density: the ratio of the weight of a given volume of a solution to the weight of the same volume of water.

Specification (purchase) – A concise description of the weight, size, and other quality factors required for a specific item.

Specimen - A sample used for analysis and diagnosis.

Specimen kit – A container used for collecting specimens.

Spectrophotometer - An instrument used to determine the concentration of a solution by measuring the light transmitted or absorbed by the solution.

Sperm - Male sex cell.

Spermatozoan - Male reproductive cell; gamete.

Sphincter - Muscular ring that regulates the size of an opening.

Sphygmomanometer - A medical device comprised of an inflatable cuff to restrict blood flow and a mercury or mechanical manometer to measure the individual's blood pressure; also called blood pressure meter.

Spinal drape - Covering for the spine during surgery or spinal anesthesia.

Spinal puncture - The removal of cerebrospinal fluid (CSF) for diagnostic purposes; also called lumbar puncture or spinal tap.

Spinal stenosis - Narrowing of areas in the lumbar (back) or cervical (neck) spine that causes pressure on the spinal cord or one or more of the spinal nerves.

Spinal tap tray - A collection of instruments and supplies for use in puncture of the spine to obtain spinal fluid for analysis and to determine the pressure within the cerebrospinal cavities.

Spirillum - Spiral-shaped bacterium of the genus spirillum; chief pathogens causing rat bite fever and Asiatic cholera.

Spirochete - Slender, corkscrew-like or spiral-shaped bacteria found on man, animals, plants and in soil and water; moves in a waving and twisting motion; some cause disease.

Spirometer – A medical device which tests lung function by measuring lung air volumes and flow rates.

Spleen - Lymphoid organ in the upper left region of the abdomen.

Splenectomy – A surgical procedure to remove the spleen.

Splint - An appliance designed for immobilization of fractures or ligamentous injuries.

Split-shift (work schedule) – A schedule plan in which employees work during two separate time periods in the same day.

Split thickness skin graft (STSG) – A graft that includes two layers of skin: the full epidermal skin layer and part of the dermal skin layer.

Sponge - Gauze material used to absorb blood and other fluids.

Sporadic disease – A disease that occurs in neither an endemic nor epidemic.

Spore – A microorganism capable of forming a thick wall around itself to enable survival in adverse conditions; a resistant form of bacterium.

Spore strip – A paper strip impregnated with a known population of microorganisms that meets the definition of biological indicator.

Sporicidal - Describing an agent's ability to kill spores.

Sporicide – An agent which destroys spores.

Sputum - Expectorate; discharge of bronchial fluids or substances.

Spunbond-meltblown-spunbond (SMS) – A non-woven packaging material which is the most popular flat wrap.

ss – One-half.

SS – Short stay.

Staff specialists – Technical advisors who provide advice to line managers about their areas of expertise.

Staffing plan – A scheduling tool used to determine the number of labor hours required for each position and each shift to meet processing requirements while maintaining quality standards.

Stain – A substance used to color cells or tissues to differentiate them for microscopic examination and study; see gram stain.

Stakeholder – A person with a vested interest in the successful outcome of a product or service; example: CSSD department stakeholders include operating room personnel and patients.

Standard - Uniform method of defining basic parameters for processes, products, services, and measurement.

Standardization - Being made uniform.

Standardized interview – An applicant interview that uses the same questions and identical question sequence to discern differences between interviewees' responses; same as structured interview.

Standard of care (to patients) – The concept that healthcare facilities must help patients by doing all that is reasonable and in good judgment.

Standard precautions – Using appropriate barriers to prevent transmission of infectious organisms from contact with blood and all other body fluids, non-intact skin, and mucous membranes; applies to all patients, regardless of diagnosis or presumed infectious status.

Standards (AAMI) - Recommendations representing a consensus of AAMI members that provide guidance to device manufacturers about design, performance, labeling, and other factors applicable to instruments they manufacture.

Standards (regulatory) - Comparison benchmarks mandated by a governing agency and, if not complied with, may cause a facility to be in violation and liable for legal penalty.

Standards (The Joint Commission) – Measures that address an organization's level of performance in key functional areas including patent rights and treatment and infection control.

Standards (voluntary) - Comparison benchmarks strongly recommended by a governing agency or professional organization that provide recommendations and guidelines for patient care.

Standing order – An agreement made between a purchaser and a vendor that the same quantity of specified product is required each time a delivery is made.

Stapedectomy - Surgical removal of the stapes in the ear.

Staphylococci - Gram-positive bacteria which grow in grape-like clusters.

Stasis - Stoppage in the normal flow of fluids such as blood, lymph, urine, or contents of the digestive tract.

STAT – Abbreviation for the Latin term, "statim:" immediately or at once.

Static – A word element meaning inhibition of bacterial growth or reproduction.

Statute - Written and enforceable law enacted by a governing body.

STD – Sexually transmitted disease.

Steam purity – The degree to which steam is free of dissolved and suspended particles, water treatment chemicals, and other contaminants.

Steam quality – The weight of dry steam present in a mixture of dry saturated steam and entrained (suspended) water.

Steam - Water vapor at 212°F (100°C) or above.

STEL – Short-term excursion limit.

Stenosis - Narrowing of a duct or canal.

Stereotactic instrument - An apparatus attached to the head; used to localize precisely an area in the brain by means of coordinates related to intracerebral structures.

Stereotype – A preconceived belief or opinion about a group of people applied to every person in that group.

Sterilant/sterilization agent - Physical or chemical substance or combination of substances that has sufficient microbicidal activity to achieve sterility under defined conditions.

Sterile - Completely devoid of all living microorganisms.

Sterile field – The immediate environment around a trauma site or surgical incision; includes all materials in contact with the wound, gowns worn by the surgical team (front panel from chest to the level of the operative field and sleeve from the cuff to two inches above the elbow), patient drapes (area adjacent to the wound), and table covers (top surface).

Sterile storage area – The area of a healthcare facility designed to store clean and sterile supplies and to protect them from contamination.

Sterile technique - Practices designed to prevent microbial contamination.

Sterility (event-related) – The concept that items are considered sterile unless the integrity of the packaging is compromised or suspected of being compromised regardless of the sterilization date; also called ERS (event-related sterility).

Sterility (time-related) – The concept that a package is considered sterile until a specific expiration date is reached.

Sterility assurance level (SAL) – The probability of a viable microorganism being present on a product unit after sterilization.

Sterility maintenance – The process of protecting a sterile item from any event that will contaminate it.

Sterility maintenance cover - See dust cover.

Sterilization – The process by which all forms of microbial life including bacteria, viruses, spores, and fungi are completely destroyed.

Sterilization area – The location of steam sterilizers including the space for loading, queuing carts, cool-down, and unloading carts.

Sterilization process monitor – A physical/chemical device used to monitor one or more parameters to detect failures due to packaging, loading, and/or sterilizer functioning. These devices cannot guarantee, assure, or prove sterilization; they measure physical conditions.

Sterilization wrap – A device intended to enclose another medical device to be sterilized by a healthcare provider and to maintain sterility of the enclosed device until used.

Sterilizer - Equipment to sterilize medical devices, equipment, and supplies by direct exposure to sterilizing agent.

Sterilizer (ethylene oxide) - Sterilizing equipment that utilizes ethylene oxide under defined conditions of gas concentration, temperature, and percent relative humidity.

Sterilizer (steam) - Sterilizing equipment that uses saturated steam under pressure as the sterilant.

Sterilizer (steam, dynamic-air-removal type) – A steam sterilizer in which air is removed from the chamber and the load by means of pressure and vacuum excursions or by means of steam flushes and pressure pulses.

Sterilizer (low temperature) - equipment to process heat sensitive devices using sterilant such as eto, hydrogen peroxide, plasma or ozone.

Sternal - Pertaining to the sternum.

Sternal puncture - Procedure used to obtain a sample of bone marrow from the sternum.

Sternoid - Resembling the sternum.

Sternotomy – An incision through the sternum to expose tissue.

Sternum - Breast bone.

Stethoscope - An acoustic medical device used to transmit low-volume sounds such as heartbeat or intestinal, venous, or fetal sounds; generally comprised of two earpieces connected by flexible tubing to a diaphragm placed against the skin of the patient.

Stilet – A small, sharp, pointed instrument used to probe, stabilize needles or catheters for insertion and to remove obstructions from lumens of needles and tubes.

Stock out (inventory) – The condition that occurs when reusable or consumable inventory items required to provide healthcare services to patients are not available.

Stockless inventory - A distribution method that involves the manufacturer or vendor delivering items as they are needed; very little inventory is kept in the facility; also called supplier-managed inventory or consignment inventory.

Stoma – Artificially-created opening.

Stomach – The pouch that serves as a reservoir for food that has been consumed.

Stomatitis - Inflammation of the mouth.

Stomatogastric - Pertaining to the stomach and the mouth.

Stopcock – An instrument used to regulate the flow of fluid through a tube or pipe.

Storing – The process of holding items under optimal storage conditions until they are needed for production or use.

Strabismus - A weakness of the eye muscle.

Strain – A specific specimen or culture of a given species; also an injury to a muscle in which the muscle fiber tears as the result of overstretching in the muscle.

Strategic planning – The process of identifying an organization's long-term goals and then determining the best approaches to achieve them; initiated by top-level administrators, and specific departments develop goals that facilitate attainment of the broader goals.

Strategic project planning team – Those members of the CSSD and other facility departments along with representatives of external regulatory, consultant, and other organizations who work together to plan facility construction projects.

Steam sterilizer – A device used for complete destruction of microorganisms by subjecting them to saturated steam under pressure at a particular temperature for a specified period.

Streptococci - Bacteria that divide to form chains; members of the genus streptococcus which are Gram-positive, chain-forming bacteria.

Stretcher - A narrow, bed-like device with wheels used for transporting a person from one point to another.

Strike-through - Penetration of liquid or microorganism through a fabric.

Stringer- Device to organize ring handle instruments inside the sterilization tray.

STSG – Split thickness skin graft

Stylet – See stilet.

Sub-account – A detailed list of expenses associated with a major category of expenses. For example, labor expense sub-accounts indicate costs for salaries, wages, overtime, benefits, and other categories of compensation.

Sub-contractor – An individual or business that signs a contract to perform part of the project that is the responsibility of the contractor.

Subcutaneous - Under the skin.

Subdural tray - A collection of instruments and supplies used to relieve intracranial pressure.

Sublingual - Pertaining to under the tongue.

Subordinate – An employee who is supervised by someone in a higher organizational position.

Subpoena – A court order for a witness to appear at a specific time and place to testify and/or to produce documents.

Suction catheter – A device used for removal of liquids or secretions such as those of the respiratory tract.

Suction devices - Surgical instruments used to extract blood from a surgical site.

Suction pump – A device that provides suction by alternating the expansion and contraction of air within a cylinder at regular intervals; also called aspirator.

Suffix (word element) – A word element that comes after the root word element.

SUD – Single-use device.

Sudden infant death syndrome (SIDS) – A medical term that describes the sudden death of an infant that remains unexplained after all known and possible causes have been carefully ruled out.

Summons (legal) – A document issued by the court when a lawsuit is filed that contains basic information about the plaintiff and defendant.

Superheated steam - Steam at a temperature which exceeds that of saturated steam at the same pressure; dry steam: the condition of steam when its temperature is too high relative to its pressure in a steam table.

Superheating – The condition that arises when steam is at a temperature which exceeds that of saturated steam at the same pressure.

Superior - Above; in a higher position.

Superordinate – The person or position to whom someone reports.

Supervisor – One who directs the work of entry-level employees.

Super-user – A person with unlimited access privileges to a computerized information system.

Supine - Lying on the back.

Supplier (vendor) – A business that sells items to a healthcare facility.

Supply chain – A coordinated system of organizations, people, activities, information, and resources used to move a product or service from the vendor to the customer. Activities in the supply chain change raw materials and components into finished products delivered to the end customer.

Supply Processing and Distribution Department (SPDD) – See Central Sterile Supply Department.

Suprapubic urinary drainage - Use of a catheter (bendable rubber tube) inserted directly from the abdomen into the urinary bladder to drain urine.

Surface tension – The contractile surface force of a liquid which makes it tend to assume a spherical form; for example, to form a meniscus; also exists at the junction of two liquids.

Surfactant – A surface-acting agent that lowers the surface tension of a liquid so it can penetrate deeper and prevent debris from being re-deposited on the item to which the soil was attached; three types: nonionic, anionic and cationic.

Surgery - A room or department where surgeons perform operative procedures.

Surgery block time schedule – The days and times during which specific surgical procedures are normally performed. For example, orthopedic procedures may be performed every morning between 7:00AM and 2:00PM.

Surgical drape – A device made of natural or synthetic materials used as a protective patient covering. Its purpose is to isolate a site of surgical incision from microbial and other contamination.

Surgical equipment - Nonexpendable apparatus used during surgical procedures; for example operating tables, back tables, etc. They are differentiated from surgical instruments which are usually hand-held and used in the immediate operative field.

Surgical gloves - Gloves designed for natural fit, sensitivity, and comfort necessary for complicated procedures.

Surgical gown - Devices worn by operating room personnel during surgical procedures to protect the patient and operating room staff from the transfer of microorganisms, body fluids, and particulate matter.

Surgical prep - Preparation of the operative site for surgery.

Surgical technologist – A person who assists in surgical operations under the supervision of surgeons, registered nurses, or other surgical personnel; also called scrub and surgical or operating room technician.

Surgical towel – An absorbent product, typically made of cotton, intended to be used in a patient-care procedure.

Surveillance – The process of monitoring closely.

Susceptible host (chain of infection) -A person or animal that lacks the ability to resist infection by an infectious agent.

Suspension – A mixture that will separate unless shaken.

Suture (joint) – A joint in which bone surfaces are closely united; for example, skull.

Suture (stitch) – A stitch used in surgery to bring parts together.

Suture removal set - A collection of instruments and supplies used to remove stitches.

Suturing -The process of securing skin edges together.

Swab - A wad of absorbent material, like cotton, wound around a small stick.

Symbiosis - Living together or close association of two dissimilar organisms with mutual benefit.

Symptom - Subjective disturbance due to disease.

Synapse – The junction between two neurons or between a neuron and an effecter.

Syndrome – A group of symptoms characteristic of a disorder.

Synergism – The action of an inactive material that improves or increases the action of an active material; case in which the sum of the actions of two or more active materials mixed together is greater than the sum of their individual actions.

Synovial - Pertaining to a thick lubricating fluid found in joints, bursae, and tendon sheaths; pertaining to freely movable (diarthrotic) joint.

Synthesis - The combining of elements to produce a compound.

Synthetic - Produced by chemical synthesis rather than of natural origin.

Syringe - A device in various sizes used to inject or withdraw fluids.

System – A group of organs that work together to carry out a specific activity.

Systems integration – The process of physically or functionally linking different computing systems and software functions.

Systole – The contraction phase of the cardiac cycle.

T – Temperature.

T – Thoracic.

T & A – Tonsil and adenoids.

t cell – A lymphocyte active in immunity that matures in the thymus gland; destroys foreign cells directly; T lymphocyte.

T&C – Type and cross match.

t.i.d. – Three times a day.

Table-top sterilizer – A compact steam sterilizer with a chamber volume of not more than two cubic feet that generates its own steam with distilled or deionized water added by the user.

tabs - Tablets.

Tachycardia – A heart rate over 100 beats per minute.

TAH - Total Abdominal Hysterectomy.

Tap water - Treated water that is acceptable for drinking.

Targeting zero - An initiative emphasizing that every healthcare facility should be working toward a goal of zero healthcare-associated infections.

Tarsals - Ankle bones.

TASS - Toxic anterior segment syndrome; inflammatory reaction to agents entering the eye.

TB – Tuberculosis.

Technical quality control indicators - Process control measures used to assure that planned technical conditions within sterilizers and aerators are met.

Technique - A method of accomplishing a desired aim.

Telecommunication system – A communication process that uses a transmitter, receiver, and physical or wireless connection to communicate.

Telemetry - Medical equipment that monitors the remote measurement and transmission of patient data via a telecommunications system to a provider's site for analysis and decision making.

TEMP – Temperature.

Temporomandibular joint – Joint of the jaw.

Tendinitis - Inflammation of the tendon.

Tendon – A cord of fibrous tissue that attaches a muscle to a bone.

Tensile strength – The amount of tensile (stretching) stress a material can withstand before breaking or failing.

Teratogen – Agents such as alcohol or thalidomide that can cause birth defects or the malfunction of an embryo.

Terminate – to end something, such as to terminate employment.

Terminal ("dumb") – A terminal with a display monitor, keyboard and, perhaps, a mouse, but with no processing ability or hard drive.

Terminal disinfection – The disinfection of a room after it has been vacated by a patient.

Terminal emulation – A process by which a specially-equipped personal computer can communicate with a mainframe computer.

Terminal infection – An infection with streptococci or other pathogenic bacteria that occurs during the course of a chronic disease which causes death.

Terminal sterilization – The process of sterilizing a packaged item.

Terminology - Specific terms used in a specialized field.

Terms and conditions (purchasing) – General provisions that apply to a supplier's price quotations and a buyer's purchase orders regardless of the specific products or services being purchased.

Test - A means of analysis or diagnosis.

Testes - Male reproductive glands that form and secrete sperm and several fluid elements in semen.

Testosterone – The male sex hormone produced in the testes; promotes the development of sperm cells and maintains secondary sex characteristics.

Tetanus – An infectious disease caused by a bacterium (Clostridium tetani); lockjaw.

Tetany - Muscle spasms due to abnormal calcium metabolism as in parathyroid deficiency.

The Joint Commission – An independent, not-for-profit organization that is the most predominant standard-setting and accrediting body in health care in the United States.

Theft – The act of unlawfully taking another's property.

Therapy - Treatment of disease.

Thermal disinfection - Use of heat to kill all organisms except spores.

Thermal equilibrium – The condition in which all parts of a system have reached the same temperature; in a steam autoclave or hot-air oven, when the temperature throughout the entire load is the same.

Thermocouple - A device composed of two lengths of wire, each of which is made of a different homogenous metal; used to measure temperature changes by connecting a potentiometer or pyrometer into the thermocouple circuit.

Thermolabile - Easily altered or decomposed by heat.

Thermometer - An instrument used to determine temperature.

Thermophiles (bacteria) - Bacteria that grow best at a temperature of 122°F – 158°F (50°C – 70°C).

Thermostable - Not easily affected by moderate heat.

Thermostatic - Controlled by temperature.

Thoracentesis - The surgical puncture and drainage of the chest cavity for diagnosis of lung disease or removal of fluid from the thorax.

Thoracic - Pertaining to the chest.

Thoracic surgery - Operative care of patients with conditions within the chest including coronary artery disease, lung cancer, esophageal cancer, heart valve and major vessel abnormalities.

Thoracotomy - The surgical incision of the chest wall.

Thorax - Chest; thoracic.

Threshold limit value (TLV) – TLVs refer to airborne concentrations of substances and represent conditions under which it is believed that nearly all workers may be repeatedly exposed day after day without adverse health effects.

Threshold limit value - ceiling (TLV-C) - The concentration that should not be exceeded during any part of the working exposure. If instantaneous monitoring is not feasible, the TLV-C can be assessed by sampling over a 15-minute period except for substances that may cause immediate irritation when exposures are short.

Threshold limit value-short term exposure limit (TLV-STEL) – A 15-minute TWA exposure which should not be exceeded at any time during a workday even if the 8-hour TWA is within the TLV-TWA. Exposure above the TLV-TWA up to the STEL should not be longer than 15 minutes and should not occur more than four times per day. There should be at least 60 minutes between successive exposures in this range.

Threshold limit value-time-weighted Average (TLV-TWA) - The time weighted average concentration for a normal 8-hour workday and a 40-hour work week to which nearly all workers may be repeatedly exposed, day after day, without adverse effect.

Thrombocyte – A blood platelet that participates in clotting.

Thrombus – A blood clot within a vessel.

Throughput – Output relative to input; the rate at which something can be processed.

Thumb forceps – A tweezer-like instrument with a smooth tip; usually held between the thumb and index finger; used to grasp objects.

Thyroid - Endocrine gland in the neck.

TIA – Transient ischemic attack.

Tib – Tibia.

TIBC – Total iron-binding capacity.

Tibia – A large bone in lower leg.

Time-weighted average (TWA) - The employee's average airborne exposure in any 8-hour work shift of a 40-hour work week which shall not be exceeded; see also threshold limit value.

Tincture – A liquid in which a chemical is dissolved in alcohol.

Tissue – A group of similar cells that performs a specialized function.

Tissue culture - Cultivation of tissue cells in vitro.

Tissue dissection – The process of cutting apart or separating tissue in a surgical procedure.

Tissue forceps – A tweezer-like instrument with teeth to grasp tissue.

Titer – The concentration of infective microbes in a medium; the amount of one substance to correspond with given amount of another substance.

Titration - Volumetric determination against standard solutions of known strength.

TLV - Threshold limit value.

TLV-C - Threshold limit value-ceiling.

TLV-STEL - Threshold limit value - short term exposure limit.

TLV-TWA - Threshold limit value-time-weighted average.

TMJ – Temporomandibular joint.

Tolerance – The ability to withstand or endure without ill effects.

Tongue depressor – An instrument used to depress the tongue for examination of the mouth and throat.

Tonsil - Mass of lymphoid tissue in the pharynx region.

Total abdominal hysterectomy (TAH) – A hysterectomy that involves making an incision in the abdominal wall.

Total acquisition costs - All costs incurred by a facility to purchase a specific supply or equipment item from the point of authorization through its disposal.

Total parenteral nutrition (TPN) – A concentrated solution that provides all daily nutritional requirements; supplied through a central venous catheter.

Total quality improvement (TQI) – The concept of measuring the current output of a process or procedure and then modifying it to increase the output, increase efficiency, and/or increase effectiveness.

Total quality management (TQM) – The quality management approach based on participation of all members aimed at long-term success through customer satisfaction and benefits to all members of the organization and society.

Tourniquet - A band used to constrict blood flow in the veins.

Toxemia - General intoxication caused by absorption of bacterial products, usually toxins, formed at a local source of infection.

Toxic anterior segment syndrome (TASS) – A noninfectious inflammation of the anterior (front) segment of the eye that is a complication of cataract or other anterior segment eye surgery.

Toxic - Poisonous.

Toxin - Poison; poisonous substance produced by and during the growth of certain pathogenic bacteria.

Toxoid - Detoxified toxin that produces specific antibodies; neutralized specific toxins used to immunize against bacteria that produce specific toxins.

TPA – Tissue plasminogen activator.

TPN – Total parenteral nutrition.

TPR – Temperature, pulse and respirations.

TQI - Total quality improvement.

TQM - Total quality management.

Tracer methodology (The Joint Commission) – The use of actual clients, patients, or residents as the framework for assessing standards compliance. Individual tracers follow the experience of care for individuals through the entire health care process.

Trachea - Windpipe.

Tracheostomy – A surgical opening into the trachea to introduce a tube through which the patient may breathe; also called tracheotomy. The opening itself may also be called a tracheostomy.

Tracheotomy catheter - A device used for tracheal aspirations.

Tracheotomy mask - A covering used for providing oxygen and moisture through a tracheostomy.

Tracheotomy tube - A device used to provide a continuous artificial airway.

Traction - A pulling force exerted on a skeletal structure by a special device.

Trainer/mentor assessment – A process to determine issues not related to task competencies that impact an employee's performance.

Training (competency-based) – Training that provides each employee with the skills and knowledge to perform work according to basic standards identified by the trainers.

Training (formal) – The process of developing the knowledge, skills, and attitudes necessary for staff members to perform required job tasks.

Training (informal) – The underlying behaviors that tell trainees how things are really done.

Training lesson – The information to be presented in a single session of a training plan; each lesson contains training objectives and indicates the content and methods required to master the content.

Training plan – A description of the structure (overview) and sequence of an entire training program.

Trait - Characteristic.

Transducer – A device that converts energy from one form to another; an ultrasonic transducer changes high-frequency electrical energy into high-frequency sound waves.

Transformational (leadership style) – A leadership approach in which leaders interact with employees in a way that permits both the leaders and their associates to raise one another to a higher level of motivation.

Transfusion - The process of injecting the blood or fluid of one person into the blood vessels of another person.

Transient ischemic attack (TIA) - A "warning stroke" or "mini-stroke" that produces stroke-like symptoms but no lasting damage.

Transmission – The transfer of anything such as a disease.

Transplant – The portion of a bacterial culture that has been transferred from an old pure culture to a fresh new medium; the transfer of organs from one person to another.

Transplantation - The replacement of an organ with one from another person.

Transrectal ultrasound - The use of sound waves to detect cancer. An instrument is inserted into the rectum. Waves bounce off the prostate and the pattern of the echoes produced is converted into a picture by a computer.

Transurethral microwave therapy (TMT) - An outpatient procedure to treat urinary symptoms caused by an enlarged prostate.

Transurethral resection of bladder tumor (TURBT) - A conservative surgery for bladder cancer in which a cytoscope is inserted through the urethra and into the bladder. A small tool with a wire loop at the end is inserted through the cystoscope, and a high-frequency electric current passes through the wire tool to remove and burn the cancer cells.

Transurethral resection prostate (TURP) - Removal of a portion of the prostate through the urethra.

Trauma surgery - Concerned with the treatment of wounds and injuries through surgical methods.

Trendelenburg - A supine position (one in which the patient is lying on his/her back) without flexing or extending and in which the head is higher than the feet.

Trendelenburg (reverse) – A supine position (one in which the patient is lying on his/her back) without flexing or extending and in which the feet are higher than the head.

Triage - System designed to sort out or classify emergency room patients according to severity of their injury or disease.

Tricuspid valve – The valve between the right atrium and right ventricle of the heart.

Triggering event (attitude) – A situation that helps to promote the development of an attitude about a person, situation, or object.

Trocar - A device used to insert a cannula into a body cavity to create a drainage outlet.

TSH – Thyroid-stimulating hormone.

tsp - Teaspoon.

Tube feeding - A method used to feed liquids into the stomach.

Tuberculin – A filterable substance produced in the growth of mycobacterium tuberculosis in culture media; when injected intracutaneously in persons exposed to the tuberculosis bacillus or its products, a reaction is produced in 24 to 48 hours consisting of infiltration and hyperemia.

Tuberculocidal - Having the ability to kill tubercle bacilli.

Tuberculosis (TB) – A highly variable and communicable disease of man and some animals caused by the tubercle bacillus (Mycobacterium tuberculosis) and characterized by the formation of tubercles in the lungs or elsewhere.

Tugger (Tug) – Warehouse equipment used to move (pull or drag) heavy large items from one location to another.

TUMT - Transurethral microwave therapy.

TURBT - Transurethral resection of bladder tumor.

Turbidity - Occurs when water contains sediments or solids that, when stirred, make the water appear cloudy.

Turn around (instrumentation) – Instruments that are required for use in back-to-back or other closely-scheduled procedures.

Turnover (employee) – The replacement of one employee by another.

Turnover rate (inventory) – A calculation of the frequency with which inventory items are purchased and used; the average amount of time that products remain in inventory.

TURP – Transurethral resection of the prostate.

TWA - Time weighted average.

TVH - Total vaginal hysterectomy.

Tympanic membrane – The membrane between the external and middle ear that transmits sound waves to the bones of the middle ear; eardrum.

U

UA – Urinalysis

Ubiquitous - Present everywhere or in many places.

UCC – Uniform commercial code.

Ulcer - Area of the skin or mucous membrane in which the tissues are gradually destroyed.

Ulna - One of the two bones in the forearm.

Ulnar nerve - The ulnar nerve is the largest unprotected nerve in the human body. It travels from under the collarbone and along the inside of the upper arm. It is commonly called the "funny bone." During surgery a foam ulnar nerve protector is commonly used to prevent damaging the nerve .

Ultrasonic cleaner - A device that uses ultrasound waves in water to clean instruments by means of cavitation.

Ultrasonic nebulizer - A high-intensity ultrasound used to break up water or sterilizing agents into tiny droplets.

Ultrasonics – The physical science of acoustic waves that oscillate in approximate range of 18 to 80 KHz.

Ultrasound - The use of ultrasonic waves for diagnostic or therapeutic purposes, specifically to visualize an internal body structure, monitor a developing fetus, or generate localized deep heat to the tissues.

Ultraviolet radiation (UV) – An invisible component of sun's radiation; used infrequently to degerm air and inanimate objects.

Umbilical cord – A structure that connects the fetus with the placenta; contains vessels that carry blood between the fetus and placenta.

Umbilicus - Small scar on the abdomen that marks the former attachment of the umbilical cord to the fetus; navel.

Underpads - A soft, absorbent material placed under incontinent patients for protection of the skin.

Unicellular - Composed of a single cell.

Uniform Commercial Code (UCC) -- A model set of federal laws regulating commercial transactions, including banking and credit, but especially those related to the sale of goods.

Union – An organization certified by the National Labor Relations Board (NLRB) to act on behalf of employees regarding wages, benefits, working and employment conditions, and job security.

Unity of command – An organizing principle that suggests each employee should only have one supervisor.

United States Public Health Service (USPHS) - An agency that serves as the office of Surgeon General; includes agencies whose mission is to improve the public health.

Universal precautions - See standard precautions.

Universal product code (UPC) - A numeric code used to identify a specific product; commonly called barcode.

Unsanitary - Deficient in sanitation; unclean to such a degree as to be injurious to health.

UPC - Universal product code.

Upper respiratory infection (URI) - Any type of infection of the head and chest caused by a virus; a common cold.

Ureter - Tube-like structure extending from the kidneys to the urinary bladder that moves urine between these organs.

Ureteral catheter - A sterile tube passed through the urethra, the bladder, and into the ureter to remove urine from the kidney.

Urethra – A tube that discharges urine and semen.

Urethroscope – An endoscope passed up the urethra to view the state of the urethral wall and prostate gland; sometimes called a panendoscope.

URI – Upper respiratory infection.

Urimeter - A device used to collect urine and measure small amounts of output.

Urinal - A vessel for receiving urine.

Urinalysis - Chemical analysis of urine.

Urinary bag - A receptacle designed to collect urine when a catheter is in place in the bladder.

Urinary bladder – A reservoir for urine.

Urinary tract infection (UTI) - An infection that begins in the urinary system.

Urination – The passage of urine from the body; also called micturition.

Urine - Liquid waste excreted by kidneys.

Urinometer - A small hydrometer used to measure the specific gravity of urine.

Urological surgery - Concerned with medical and surgical treatment of disorders of the urinary and male reproductive systems.

Urologist - A physician who specializes in the urinary or urogenital tract.

Urology - The branch of medicine that deals with the diagnosis and treatment of diseases of the urinary tract and of the male reproductive organs.

Urostomy - An operation to create an opening from inside the body to the outside, making a new way to pass urine.

Use life (disinfectants) – The length of time or number of times used after which the efficiency of a disinfectant is diminished.

USPHS – United States Public Health Service.

Utensil – An instrument or container for domestic use; in hospitals, an item used for basic patient care such as a bedpan or washbasin.

Uterus - Female organ within which the fetus develops during pregnancy.

UTI – Urinary tract infection.

Utility room – Space used for the storage of clean or soiled materials and equipment.

UV – Ultraviolet radiation.

Uvula – A soft, fleshy, V-shaped mass that hangs from the soft palate.

V

Vaccination - Introduction of vaccine into the body.

Vaccine – A substance used to produce active immunity; usually a suspension of attenuated or killed pathogens given by inoculation to prevent a specific disease.

Vagina - Muscular canal in a female that extends from an external opening to the neck of the uterus.

Vaginal packing - Dressing material inserted into the vagina to medicate or stop vaginal bleeding.

Vaginal speculum - An instrument used for expanding the vagina to allow for visual examination of the vagina and cervix.

Vaginal tampon - A device to arrest hemorrhages or absorb secretions.

Validation - Decontamination procedures used by equipment manufacturers to obtain, record, and interpret test results required to establish that a process consistently produces a sterile product.

Value – The relationship between the prices paid to a vendor and what is received in return: product or service of required quality, helpful supplier information, and appropriate service.

Value analysis – The process of analyzing physician-preferred items to consider alternative costs, reimbursement, and strategic initiative concerns; the study of the relationship of design, function and cost of a product, material, or service.

Value-based purchasing (Medicare) – A Medicare payment system that links payment to providers that deliver high quality, efficient clinical care.

Valve – A structure that prevents fluid from flowing backward as in the heart, veins, and lymphatic vessels.

Vancomycin resistant enterococcus (VRE) – Enterococcus bacteria that are no longer sensitive to vancomycin; transmission can occur either by direct contract or indirectly by hands.

Vapor – A substance in the gaseous state that is usually a liquid or solid.

Vapor pressure – The pressure exerted by the molecules of a specific vapor.

Vaporizer - Medical equipment that produces vapor from volatile anesthetic agents such as ether, chloroform, or halothane. Gases are blown through, over the surface, or over a wick of the volatile liquids to produce vapor. Vaporizers usually fit on the back of the anesthesia machine so that the gas mixtures from the flow meters can pass through and collect the vapor.

Variable costs – Costs that change in relation to the value of processing output in the Central Service department; for example, waged labor and supplies.

Variance (inventory) – The difference between the amount of a supply that should be available (from records) and the amount that is available (from physical count) when a perpetual inventory system is used.

Varicella - Chickenpox.

Varicose - Pertaining to an unnatural swelling; for example, varicose veins.

Variola - Smallpox.

Vas deferens – The duct that transfers sperm from the epididymus to the seminal vesicle.

Vascular surgery - Concerned with the surgical treatment of disorders of the blood vessels.

Vasectomy - Excision of the vas deferens or a portion of the vas deferens to produce sterility in the male.

Vasoconstriction - Decrease in the diameter of a blood vessel.

Vasodilatation - Increase in the diameter of a blood vessel.

VAT—Video-assisted thoracotomy.

VBP – Value-based purchasing (Medicare).

VD - Venereal disease.

Vector - Carrier of pathogenic microorganisms from one host to another; for example: flies, fleas, and mosquitoes.

Vegetative bacteria – Non-spore-forming bacteria or spore-forming bacteria in a non-sporulating state.

Vegetative stage - State of active growth of microorganisms as opposed to resting or spore stages.

Veins - Vessels that carry blood back to the heart.

Vena cava - One of two large veins that carry blood into the right atrium of the heart.

Vendor – A business that sells products or services to the healthcare facility.

Vendor-managed inventory – A service in which a vendor stocks and maintains a facility's inventory to agreed-upon levels and then issues a monthly (or other time period) invoice for all items used.

Venereal disease (VD) – A disease acquired through sexual activity.

Venipuncture - Entry into a vein with a needle.

Venous - Relating to vein or veins.

Venous pressure – A measure of the pressure of the blood within the peripheral veins.

Vent – Ventricle; also refers to a ventilator.

Ventilation - Movement of air into and out of the lungs.

Ventilator (respiratory) - Medical equipment or a breathing machine for providing assisted or artificial ventilation of the lungs. It can be a resuscitator for emergency use, a body respirator, or lung ventilator.

Ventral - Toward the front or belly surface; anterior.

Ventricles - The two lower chambers of the heart.

Ventricular fibrillation (Vfib) - A condition in which the heart's electrical activity becomes disordered.

Ventricular septal defect (VSD) - A defect in the septum between the right and left ventricle.

Ventricular tachycardia (VT) –A fast heart beat (usually over 100 beats per minute) caused by disease or injury.

Venule – A very small vein that collects blood from the capillaries.

Verbal abuse – Abusive behavior that involves the use of language.

Verification - Decontamination procedures used to confirm that the validation undertaken by the equipment manufacturer is applicable to the specific setting.

Vertebra - One of the bones of the spinal column.

Vertebral arch - A circle of bone around the canal through which the spinal cord passes.

Vertebral column – A series of 33 irregularly shaped bones called vertebrae; also called backbone, spine or spinal column.

Vesicle – A small sac or blister filled with fluid.

Vfib – Ventricular fibrillation.

Viable - Living; having the ability to multiply.

Video-assisted thoracotomy (VAT) – A procedure to evaluate and biopsy within the pleural space and at the pulmonary hilum (depression on the surface of the lung).

Virology - Study of virus and viral diseases.

Virucidal - Describing an agent's ability to kill viruses.

Virucide – An agent that destroys or inactivates viruses.

Virulence - Capacity of microorganisms to produce disease; power of an organism to overcome defenses of the host.

Virus - One of a group of minute infectious agents that grows only in living tissues or cells.

Virus (computer) – A computer program that copies itself and infects and disrupts the operation of other computers without the users' knowledge.

Viscera - Organs in the ventral body cavities (especially the abdominal organs).

Vision – An abstract idea about what the healthcare facility or CSSD would be like if it was ideal.

VIT—Vitrectomy.

Vital - Characteristic of life; necessary for life; pertaining to life.

Vital signs (VS) - Measurements of the body's most basic functions: body temperature, pulse rate, respiration rate (rate of breathing), and blood pressure (not considered a vital sign but often measured with vital signs).

Vitrectomy (VIT) - Removal of the vitreous humor from the eyeball.

Vitreous humor - Fluid-filled compartment that gives shape to the eye.

Voice over internet protocol (VOIP) – A transmission technology that allows voice communication over the internet.

Voluntary reduction (hours) – A process in which employees voluntarily reduce their working hours and compensation for a specified time; typically used as a layoff alternative.

VRE - Vancomycin resistant enterococcus.

VS – Vital signs.

VSD – Ventricular septal defect.

VT – Ventricular tachycardia.

W

Wage – Pay based on the amount of time (usually hours) worked on the job.

Wage and salary survey – A local or nationwide benchmark report of market pay data for jobs used to evaluate an organization's current pay structure and for future compensation planning.

Wall suction unit - A mechanical suction device that must be attached to a wall suction (vacuum) outlet for power.

Warranty – A guarantee or an assurance from a seller to the buyer that the goods or property is or shall be as represented.

Washer/decontaminator - A mechanical device used to wash bedpans, glassware, instruments, basins and trays commonly used in the decontamination process.

Washer/sterilizer - A mechanical device designed to wash, disinfect, and sterilize instruments and metal ware; most commonly used in the decontamination process.

Washers - Automated equipment used to clean, decontaminate, or disinfect (low, intermediate, or low-level) and dry medical devices.

Waste – Resources or human efforts that are consumed without meaningful purpose.

WBC – White blood cell.

Webinar – A workshop or lecture delivered over the world-wide-web.

Wet pack – Containers with moisture after the sterilization process is completed.

Wetting agent – A substance that reduces the surface tension of a liquid and allows the liquid to penetrate or spread more easily across the surface of a solid.

Wetting power - Reduction of the water surface tension which allows the water to run or spread evenly over the surface.

Whipple procedure - A type of surgery used to treat pancreatic cancer. The surgeon removes the head of the pancreas, the duodenum, a portion of the stomach, and other nearby tissues.

Whistle blower program (OSHA) – Legal requirements that protect workers from negative employment actions that occur when employees report to or cooperate with OSHA concerning workplace safety violations.

White blood cell (WBC) - Blood cells that engulf and digest bacteria and fungi.

WHO – World Health Organization.

Wicking material – An approved absorbent material that allows for air removal, steam penetration and that facilitates drying.

Wide area network (WAN) – A set of widely separated computers that are connected together.

Willful misconduct – Any action taken consciously and willfully by an employee that is deliberately malicious or violates a facility policy.

Witness – Someone with first-hand or expert evidence who testifies under oath in a trial or deposition; see "deposition."

Word elements - Parts of a word.

Work flow – The logical and sequential progression of how work tasks should be done and how they should relate to each other.

Work flow (optimization) – The management of a work process in a way that enables employees to perform their tasks efficiently and effectively while eliminating non-productive steps.

Work flow chart – A graphical representation of the steps in a work process. The flow chart's elements are linked with arrows to show the direction of the process flow.

Work hardening – A work-oriented therapy to help employees injured on the job to bridge the gap between completion of physical or occupational therapy and their return to the workplace.

Work practice controls - Controls that reduce the likelihood of exposure by altering the manner in which a task is performed; for example, prohibiting recapping needles with a two-handed technique.

Work simplification – The process of making a job easier and/or simpler to perform.

Work station – The area including applicable equipment and necessary tools and supplies where an employee performs specific work tasks.

Worker's compensation claim – A payment request under a state law that issues cash payments and provides medical care to employees who are injured or disabled during the course of their employment.

Workers' compensation (insurance) – Insurance maintained by employers to benefit employees who become ill or are injured on the job.

Working capital – The funds an organization has available to conduct its daily activities; the amount by which current assets exceed current liabilities.

Workplace violence – Assaults (threats or attempts to strike another) and other violent acts that occur in or are related to the workplace that involve a substantial risk of physical or emotional harm to individuals or damage to the organization's resources or capabilities.

Work-related musculoskeletal disorder (WMSD) - An injury to or disorder of the musculoskeletal system where exposure to workplace risk factors may have contributed to the disorder's development or aggravated a pre-existing condition.

Wound - An injury to the body.

Wound V.A.C. Therapy - Provides negative pressure wound therapy by using controlled suction to close large wounds and to promote faster healing.

Writing style – The manner in which a writer addresses a topic while writing about it; helps to reveal the writer's personality or "voice."

Written warning – Written documentation given to an employee describing specific disciplinary infractions such as frequent tardiness or failure to follow policies. Written warnings clearly state the issue, identify what is needed to correct the problem, and indicate the possible consequences if improvements are not made.

X

X-ray - Radiation of extremely short wave length that can penetrate opaque substances and affects photographic plates and fluorescent screens.

Y

Yankauer suction tip - A suction tip with a large opening surrounded by a bulbous head and is designed to allow effective suction without damaging surrounding tissue; used to suction oropharyngeal secretions to prevent aspiration.

Yeasts - Any of several unicellular fungi of the genus, Saccharomyces, which reproduce by budding.

Z

Zero-tolerance (harassment policy) – A policy that permits no amount of leniency regarding harassing behavior.

Glossary of Regulation and Standard Setting Government Agencies and Voluntary Organizations

Central Service is affected by regulations issued by several governmental (regulatory) agencies and by standards recommended by numerous voluntary organizations. Their purpose is to protect the health and well-being of patients, healthcare facility employees, and others. This glossary provides a review of the agencies and organizations that most impact the policies and procedures of Central Service Departments. Note: there may also be state and local governmental agencies that develop and monitor regulations of concern to central service personnel.

Centers for Disease Control and Prevention (CDC)
http://www.cdc.gov

Role: promotes health and quality of life by preventing and controlling disease, injury and disability, and by responding to health emergencies.

Department of Transportation (DOT)
http://www.dot.gov

Role: enforces laws relating to healthcare including the transportation of medical wastes including minimally processed instrumentation for repair and labeling, and the transportation of hazardous and radioactive wastes.

Environmental Protection Agency (EPA)
http://www.epa.gov

Role: creates and enforces laws relating to cleaner water, air, and land. Two major acts that affect Central Service are The Federal Insecticide, Fungicide, and Rodenticide Act (FIFRA), and the 1990 Clean Air Acts Amendments.

Food and Drug Administration (FDA)
http://www.fda.gov

Role: ensures that foods, cosmetics, human and veterinary drugs, biological products, medical devices, and electronic products emitting radiation are safe and effective. Administers pre- and post-market medical device requirements, MedWatch, medical device classifications, and medical device recalls.

Occupational Safety and Health Administration (OSHA)

http://www.osha.gov

Role: protects workers from occupationally-caused illnesses and injuries. Develops standards that relate to occupational exposure to bloodborne pathogens and guidelines for the use of ethylene oxide sterilization.

American National Standards Institute (ANSI)

http://www.ansi.org

Role: enhances the global competitiveness of U.S. business and the American quality of life by promoting and facilitating voluntary consensus standards and ensuring their integrity.

Association for the Advancement of Medical Instrumentation (AAMI)

http://www.aami.org

Role: develops Recommended Practices and Standards that are considered major resources for Central Service guidelines.

Association of periOperative Registered Nurses (AORN)

http://www.aorn.org

Role: develops nationally recognized Standards, Recommended Practices, and Guidelines for the periOperative setting.

The Association for Professionals in Infection Control and Epidemiology, Inc. (APIC)

http://www.apic.org

Role: addresses the prevention and control of infections and related outcomes.

International Standards Organization (ISO)

http://www.iso.org

Role: uses a network of National Standards Institutes to develop voluntary standards from those proposed by members such as AAMI that are based on the consensus of the entire membership.

The Joint Commission

http://www.jointcommission.org

Role: provides standards for healthcare facilities and evaluates United States healthcare organizations using on-site surveys at least every three years.

National Fire Protection Association (NFPA)

http://www.nfpa.org

Role: develops International standards to reduce the incidence of fire and other hazards. Sets standards for fire burden of all the disposable packaged items stored and used within healthcare facilities, as well as the fire standards for the patient drapes used in the Operating Room.

Society of Gastroenterology Nurses and Associates (SGNA)

http://www.sgna.org

Role: establishes standards for the effective processing of flexible endoscopes.

United States Pharmacopeia – National Formulary (USP-NF)

http://www.usp.org/uspnf

Role: creates and revises standards for medicines, dosages, forms, drug substances, and dietary supplements. Develops standards applicable to Central Service Departments that process water for irrigation.

World Health Organization (WHO)

http://www.who.org

Role: furthers international cooperation in improving health conditions by combating disease (especially key infectious diseases), and by promoting the general health of the peoples of the world.

Celsius – Fahrenheit Temperature Conversion

Use the following formula to convert Celsius readings to Fahrenheit readings:

°F = 9/5°C + 32

For example, if the Celsius reading is 37°:

°F = (9 / 5 x 37) + 32

= 66.6 + 32

= 98.6°F. (normal body temperature)

Use the following formula to convert Fahrenheit reading to Celsius readings:

°C = 5 / 9 (°F − 32)

For example, if the Fahrenheit reading is 68°:

°C = 5 / 9 (68-32)

= 5 / 9 x 36

= 20°C (a nice spring day)

Understanding Fahrenheit and Celsius

The main difference between Fahrenheit and Celsius is their relative values for both the freezing points and boiling points for water. This causes all other temperature points on the thermometer to be different as well. Celsius is considered a world standard because of its ease of use. However, many people operate on the Fahrenheit system for many applications such as weather information, cooking and sterilization parameters.

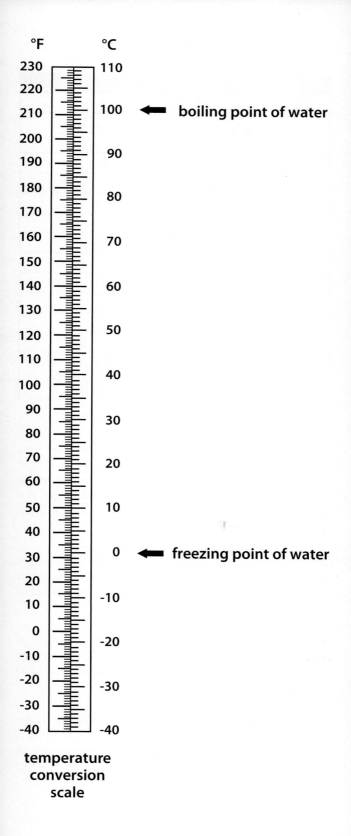

temperature
conversion
scale

Time Conversion Chart

Day am		Evening pm	
Standard	24 Hour	Standard	24 Hour
1:00 = 0100		13:00 = 1300	
2:00 = 0200		14:00 = 1400	
3:00 = 0300		15:00 = 1500	
4:00 = 0400		16:00 = 1600	
5:00 = 0500		17:00 = 1700	
6:00 = 0600		18:00 = 1800	
7:00 = 0700		19:00 = 1900	
8:00 = 0800		20:00 = 2000	
9:00 = 0900		21:00 = 2100	
10:00 = 1000		22:00 = 2200	
11:00 = 1100		23:00 = 2300	
12:00 = 1200		24:00 = 2400*	

* At the completion of the 24 hour cycle, the clock starts over at 0000 hours. Therefore midnight is sometimes referred to as 00:00 hours.

Understanding 24 Hour Times

Times are expressed using the 24-hour clock. The time begins at midnight (0000 hours) and continues. Midnight is zero hour and is written 00:00. Other times are simply the number of hours and minutes after midnight. For example, 1:00PM is displayed as 1300 because it is 13 hours past midnight.

Note: The 24 hour clock begins with 0000 hours, sometimes called 2400 hours. When spoken aloud, this is said, "twenty-four hundred hours," which is the equivalent of midnight.

Morning hours are described as follows: 1:00AM is 0100 hours, called "oh one hundred hours". The pattern continues for the morning hours until noon which is 1200 hours ("twelve hundred hours").

24 hour time continues to ascend for the afternoon hours rather than beginning a new 12-hour cycle so 1:00PM is called 1300 hours. Those numbers ascend until midnight when the 24 hour clock begins again.

pH Scale

Acidity and alkalinity are terms which describe extreme differences in a solution just as hot and cold are terms which describe extreme differences in temperature. Just as mixing hot and cold water evens out the temperature, mixing acids and bases can cancel their extreme effects. That state is described as neutral.

The pH scale indicates whether a solution is more acid or more alkaline, just as the Fahrenheit or Celsius scale is used to measure temperature. The range of the pH scale is from 0 to 14 from very acid to very alkaline. A pH of 7 is neutral. A pH less than 7 is acidic and greater than 7 is alkaline.

Each whole pH value below 7 is ten times more acidic than the next higher value. For example, a pH of 4 is ten times more acidic than a pH of 5 and a hundred times (10 X 10) more acidic than a pH of 6. This holds true for pH values above 7, each of which is ten times more alkaline (also called basic) than the next lower whole value. For example, a pH of 10 is ten times more alkaline than a pH of 9.

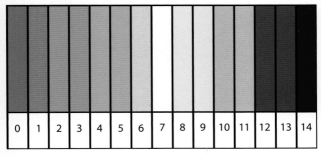

pH is used to measure acidity or alkalinity.

Acids turn litmus paper RED.

Alkalis (sometimes called bases) turn litmus paper BLUE.

Dental Wire and Suture Wire Measurements

Dental Wire and Suture Wire

The Stubs Iron Wire Gauge system (also known as the Birmingham Wire Gauge) is used in health care to measure needles and suture wires. It was originally developed for use in manufacturing, and began appearing in the healthcare setting to describe needle sizes and surgical and dental wire sizes.

Wire gauge is inversely proportional to its diameter, so the larger the gauge number, the smaller the wire diameter.

Needle Information

CSSD professionals work with many types of needles. The information below provides some information on needle terminology.

Needle – A cannula with a hub attached used primarily for injecting and aspirating fluids. Some specialty needles are designed to perform biopsies, or work in conjunction with specific instrument systems. Most needles are disposable, but reusable varieties are used for some procedures. Needle assemblies can be made from metal or plastic.

Gauge - The width or diameter of the needle is measured in gauges. The larger the gauge size number, the smaller the size of the needle. In the United States needles typically use gauge sizes from 13 to 31.

Bevel – The ground surface of a cannula, (also called needle point or needle tip).

Luer – Male or Female taper on end of a needle hub that is used to connect a needle to a syringe or other Luer fitting. Hubs can be Luer Slip (slide on) or Luer Lock (twist on).

Surgical Suture Needles – Needles designed to perform ligation processes. Surgical suture needles vary in size and style depending on the type of process they are designed to perform.

Surgical Style Needles

Many of the needles used for surgical procedures are specifically designed for a particular process. When working with surgical supply requests, CSSD professionals may encounter abbreviations that are very important to ensure that the correct needle is provided. The table below provides some common needle style abbreviations.

Common Needle Style Abbreviations

Needle Style Abbreviation	Type of Needle
BF	Blunt Intraocular Fixation
BP	Blunt Point
C	Cardiovascular
CE	Cutting Edge
CFS	Conventional for Skin
CIF	Cutting Intraocular Fixation
CP	Cutting Point
CPS	Conventional Plastic Surgery
CPX	Cutting Point Extra Large
CT	Circle Taper
CTB	Circle Taper Blunt
CTX	Circle Taper Extra Large
CTXB	Circle Taper Extra Large Blunt
CV	Cardiovascular
DC	Dura Closure
DP	Double Point
EST	Eyed Straight Taper
FN	For Tonsil
FS	For Skin
FSL	For Skin Large
FSLX	For Skin Large Extra
G	Greishaber
GS	Greishaber Spatula
KS	Keith Straight
LH	Large Half (circle)
LR	Large Retention
LS	Large Sternotomy
M	Muscle
MF	Modified Ferguson
MH	Medium Half (circle)
MO	Mayo
OPS	Ocular Plastic Surgery
OS	Orthopedic Surgery
P	Plastic
PC	Precision Cosmetic

PS	Plastic Surgery
RH	Round Half (circle)
S	Spatula
SC	Straight Cutting
SH	Small Half (circle)
ST	Straight Taper
STB	Straight Blunt
STC	Straight Cutting
STP	Straight Taper Point
Straight	Straight
TE	Three Eighths
TG	Transverse Ground
TGW	Transverse Ground Wide
TP	Taper Point
UR	Urology
URB	Urology Blunt
X or P	Exodontal (Dental)
XLH	Extra Large Half (circle)
XXLH	Extra Extra Large Half (circle)

French Catheter Scale

The French catheter scale, or "French units" (Fr), is commonly used to measure the outside diameter of catheters and other cylindrical medical instruments.

French Gauge	Diameter (mm)	Diameter (inches)
3	1	0.039
4	1.35	0.053
5	1.67	0.066
6	2	0.079
7	2.3	0.092
8	2.7	0.105
9	3	0.118
10	3.3	0.131
11	3.7	0.144
12	4	0.158
13	4.3	0.170
14	4.7	0.184
15	5	0.197
16	5.3	0.210
17	5.7	0.223
18	6	0.236
19	6.3	0.249
20	6.7	0.263
22	7.3	0.288
24	8	0.315
26	8.7	0.341
28	9.3	0.367
30	10	0.393
32	10.7	0.419
34	11.3	0.445

Common Metric Measurements
seen in CSSD

Most countries around the world have adopted the Metric measurement system. The United States has not adopted the system; however it is commonly used in healthcare. While Central Service professionals do not work with all aspects of the Metric system, they will encounter some metric terms in their work. The table below highlights common terms that CSSD professionals may encounter.

Some Common Measurements
seen in CSSD

Used to Measure	Unit	Symbol
Length,Width, Girth	millimeter centimeter meter kilometer	mm cm m km
Mass, Weight	milligram gram kilogram	mg g kg
Temperature	Degree Celsius	0C
Volume	milliliter cubic centimeter liter	mL cc L

In the Metric system the names of multiples and submultiples are formed using prefixes. Common examples include deca- (ten), hecto- (hundred), kilo- (thousand), mega- (million), and giga- (billion); deci- (tenth), centi- (hundredth), milli- (thousandth), micro- (millionth), and nano- (billionth). The prefixes centi and milli are most commonly encounted by CSSD professionals.

When writing Metric symbols it is important to remember that those symbols are case-sensitive and care must be taken to use upper and lower case letters as indicated. Changing the case of a symbol can change its meaning.

Symbol Glossary

EC REP	Authorize representative in the European community
LOT	Batch code
(biohazard symbol)	Biological Risks
REF	Catalog number
(triangle with exclamation mark)	Caution; consult accompanying documents
(open book with i)	Consult instructions for use
CONTROL	Control
(scissors)	Cut
(circle with 2 crossed out)	Do not reuse
(damaged package crossed out)	Do not use if package damaged
(sun symbol)	Keep away from heat

	Keep away from light
	Keep dry
	Lower limit of temperature
	Manufacturer
STERILE EO	Method of sterilization: ethylene oxide
STERILE R	Method of sterilization: irradiation
CONTROL −	Negative control
#	Patient ID number
	Peel
CONTROL +	Positive control
SN	Serial number
	Temperature limitation

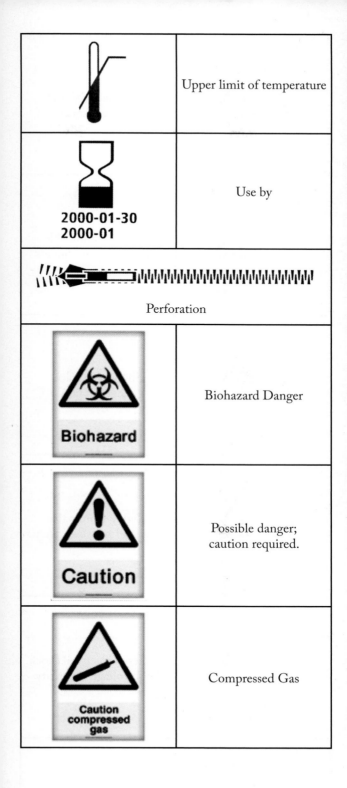

	Upper limit of temperature
2000-01-30 **2000-01**	Use by
Perforation	
Biohazard	Biohazard Danger
Caution	Possible danger; caution required.
Caution compressed gas	Compressed Gas

Caution corrosive substance	Corrosive Material may be present.
Caution hot liquids	Warning of possible contact with hot liquids.
Caution slippery surface	Slippery Surface, danger of falls.
Danger highly flammable	Highly Flammable Materials may be present.
Danger high voltage	Danger of electrical shock. High voltage electricity.
	Emergency Eyewash Station

	Emergency Fire Blanket
	Emergency Meeting Point
	Emergency Safety Shower
	Escape Route
	Products or conditions pose a danger of explosion.
	Fire Extinguisher
	Fire Extinguisher

	First Aid
High noise levels	Possible high noise levels; ear protection may be required.
Inhalation hazard	Contaminants or Vapors may be present that pose a threat of inhaled.
Laser in operation	Laser in operation. Follow required safety protocols.
Poison	Poisonous materials or vapors. Follow required safety protocols.
Radiation hazard	Radiation. Follow required safety protocols.

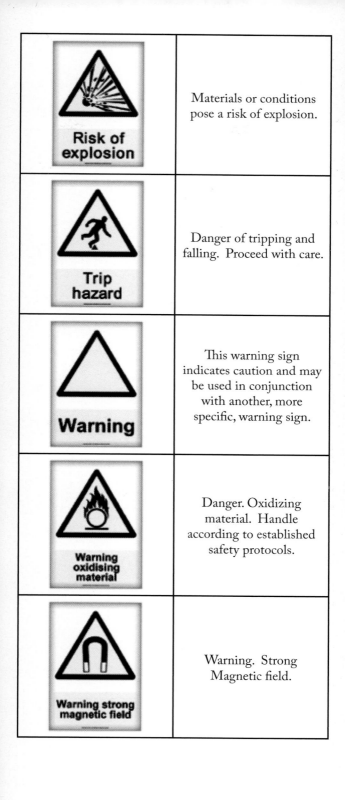

Risk of explosion	Materials or conditions pose a risk of explosion.
Trip hazard	Danger of tripping and falling. Proceed with care.
Warning	This warning sign indicates caution and may be used in conjunction with another, more specific, warning sign.
Warning oxidising material	Danger. Oxidizing material. Handle according to established safety protocols.
Warning strong magnetic field	Warning. Strong Magnetic field.